T0315186

THE
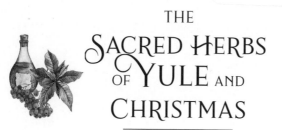

SACRED HERBS
OF YULE AND
CHRISTMAS

"This is so much more than an herbal book. Ellen has covered origins and meanings for this most wonderful time of year as well as including practical workings. Packed full with fascinating myth busters and a festive hamper brimming over with magical and medicinal herbs found and used at Yule. A comprehensive guide to working magic and connecting with the energy of the season. Highly recommended."

RACHEL PATTERSON, AUTHOR OF *A WITCH FOR EVERY SEASON*

"Amid the swirl of seasonal tastes, smells, and colors, Ellen Evert Hopman sprinkles elves and international lore in abundance. This is a delightful culinary and medicinal reference with Pagan sensibilities. Hopman's culinary recipes call for unusual herbs blended with humor and cautions in equal measure. My personal favorite is Fallen Oak Leaf Broth. What a treat!"

LYRION APTOWER, AUTHOR OF *MUSINGS & MISCELLANY*

"Winter Solstice, Yule, the longest night, shortest day; it has for centuries been held by many as a central sacred point in time. Within it is the shared experience of coming together to share in the warmth of family and community, all yearning for the return of the light. Ellen's book *The Sacred Herbs of Yule and Christmas* is stuffed full with bits of seasonal wisdom. It is a delightful gift to take with you into the dark and cold, to help warm the heart with stories and traditions, garnishing the anticipation and participation in the joy of the holiday."

LAURA WILDMAN, AUTHOR OF *WHAT'S YOUR WICCA IQ?*

"A mystical journey through a magical time of year, delving into traditions of old and magical rituals and rites to enrich the wonders of the winter season. *The Sacred Herbs of Yule and Christmas* is a highly recommended book that adds an extra sprinkling of magic and a depth of meaning to any Yuletide celebration, gathering, or personal observance."

ROXIE J. ZWICKER, AUTHOR OF
HAUNTED PORTSMOUTH AND *MAINE BOOK OF THE DEAD*

"With beautiful illustrations and many recipes, *The Sacred Herbs of Yule and Christmas* is packed full of historical information about the origins of these traditions. It would be a fun project to work through this book, especially with children, being at the same time educational without the boredom or misery often associated with learning."

LUKE EASTWOOD, AUTHOR OF *THE DRUID'S PRIMER*
AND COAUTHOR OF *KERRY FOLK TALES*

"This is a very interesting book, and Ellen Evert Hopman sure knows her stuff. I recommend *The Sacred Herbs of Yule and Christmas* to anyone interested in the Yuletide traditions. I have a number of her books and am looking to add this one to my collection."

J. T. SIBLEY, PH.D., TRADITIONAL NORSE PRACTITIONER AND
AUTHOR OF *THE WAY OF THE WISE*

"A well-developed, comprehensive, and logical presentation on the subject of herbs and seasonal celebrations for Yule and Christmas. The information is accessible for a beginner and insightful for the advanced practitioner. A well-illustrated book that can be used for both instructional and referential purposes."

AMORIC, THIRD-DEGREE ALEXANDRIAN HIGH PRIEST WITH
MORE THAN 30 YEARS OF ACTIVITY IN THE CRAFT COMMUNITY
AND CONTRIBUTOR TO *THE REAL WITCHES OF NEW ENGLAND*

THE SACRED HERBS OF YULE AND CHRISTMAS

Remedies, Recipes, Magic & Brews for the Winter Season

ELLEN EVERT HOPMAN

Destiny Books
Rochester, Vermont

Destiny Books
One Park Street
Rochester, Vermont 05767
www.DestinyBooks.com

Destiny Books is a division of Inner Traditions International

Copyright © 2023 by Ellen Evert Hopman

All rights reserved. No part of this book may be reproduced or utilized in any form
or by any means, electronic or mechanical, including photocopying, recording, or
any information storage and retrieval system, without permission in writing from the
publisher.

Note to the reader: *This book is intended to be an informational guide. The remedies,
approaches, and techniques described herein are meant to supplement, and not to be a
substitute for, professional medical care or treatment. They should not be used to treat a
serious ailment without prior consultation with a qualified health care professional.*

Cataloging-in-Publication Data for this title is available from the Library of Congress

ISBN 978-1-64411-780-4 (print)
ISBN 978-1-64411-781-1 (ebook)

Printed and bound in China by Reliance Printing Co., Ltd.

10 9 8 7 6 5 4 3 2

Text design and layout by Virginia Scott Bowman
This book was typeset in Garamond Premier Pro and Futura with Thirsk used as the
display typeface

To send correspondence to the author of this book, mail a first-class letter to the
author c/o Inner Traditions • Bear & Company, One Park Street, Rochester, VT
05767, and we will forward the communication, or contact the author directly at
www.elleneverthopman.com.

CONTENTS

PART TWO
MAGICAL AND MEDICINAL HERBS OF WINTER

ॐ

FOREWORD

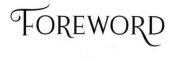

By Lucya Starza

When Ellen Evert Hopman asked me to write this foreword, I was as delighted as if I'd been handed an unexpected gift from under a tree decked with baubles and sparkling in firelight on the most magical day of the year. Peeling back the wrapping paper on that unexpected present, *The Sacred Herbs of Yule and Christmas* is exactly the kind of book I'd have wanted to find within. I'd have admired the beautiful cover, then opened the pages and started reading, enchanted by winter tales from around the world, enticed by recipes to try, and almost smelling the herbs of the season.

I've always loved Christmas and Yuletide. As a child I felt I was doubly blessed because my family celebrated both a traditional Polish Christmas Eve and an English-style Christmas Day. Although I was born in England, my father came from Poland, and I loved to spend time with my relatives on that side of the family enjoying a custom known as Wigilia. The name derives from the Latin word for vigil, and the tradition is to stay awake until midnight on December 24, which was always a treat for the very young. However, the best thing about Wigilia is the special supper. It has twelve courses, or dishes, all of them meatless, aside from fish. My aunt would cook everything from scratch, following the family recipes. The banquet started with *barszcz,* a Polish beetroot soup. There were bread rolls filled with mushrooms, pierogi stuffed with cheese, fried carp and cold herring, salad dressed with sour cream, potato and cabbage dishes, and sweets, including fruit compote, homemade jelly, poppy seed cake, and soft gingerbread.

My father's family was Catholic, so I grew up learning the Christian symbolism of Wigilia—that the vigil is for the birth of Christ, the twelve courses represent the apostles, and the pescatarian tradition honors the animals that were in the stable when Jesus was born. At the end of the meal, we shared gifts, and then my family went to midnight Mass at the local Catholic church.

I had no idea Wigilia had more ancient Pagan roots until I read in Ellen's book that the evening contains elements of the worship of an ancient Slavic winter deity known as Star Man. Star Man was traditionally a giver of gifts and was accompanied by Star Woman, who wore a crown of greenery. Today, perhaps in a nod to Star Man and Star Woman, Wigilia celebrants traditionally wait for the first star to appear on December 24 before starting their evening feast, and seeing that star is considered lucky. The twelve courses of the meal can represent the months of the year and are symbolic of wealth and abundance. I will now be honoring Star Man and Star Woman at my own Wigilia supper this December and making a wish when I see the first star twinkling in the night sky.

Ellen's book taught me about other Polish traditions, too, like that of the pudding called *kutia,* made of grain, berries, honey, nuts, and spices. The ingredients symbolize eternal life, fertility, and pleasure. The sticky pudding is shared between family members to bring unity and good fortune. According to Ellen, putting a little under a pillow, wrapped in men's trousers, is supposed to give a girl dreams of her future husband.

That intertwining of magic, lore, and kitchen craft forms the basis of Yuletide traditions around the world, new and old, near and far. This book is, ostensibly, about herbs, and Ellen is a renowned master herbalist, but we find within these pages so much more: recipes, remedies, histories, heritage. It is, perhaps, a re-homing of the holiday celebration, a reminder of the ways in which we can honor and connect with our ancestors, the ancient Gods and Goddesses, and the Spirits and energy of the land.

Ellen is the Archdruid of Tribe of the Oak, a founding member of the Order of the White Oak, and an Archdruidess of the Druid Clan of Dana. She shares here many Pagan rituals for the Yuletide season, including a complete rite for the Goddess at the Winter Solstice, originally composed in honor of the Cailleach, the winter face of the Land Goddess. As a Pagan and a Witch, I find the Winter Solstice to be a particularly special time. Ellen is, among her other attributes, a Bard of the Gorsedd of Caer Abiri, the ancient megalithic monuments at Avebury, in Wiltshire, England. It is my favorite set of stone circles. I've celebrated many Wheel of the Year festivals there, but the most memorable was when some friends and I rented a historic thatched cottage within the stones for a week around December 21. We got up before dawn to take part in the public ritual to honor the rebirth of the Sun, and then we retired indoors for food and drink, games, storytelling, and music around the fire. It felt as though we were tapping into traditions tracing back to ancient times, although with the modern convenience of a gas stove to roast our dinner and mull our wine.

That mingling of ways, old and new, is put into practice by most modern midwinter celebrations—and has, perhaps, been the tradition for all of human history. I often see people arguing on social media about which traditions and methods are the oldest or reflect the most accurate meaning of the festivities. For me, those arguments don't matter. I believe Yuletide should be a time of year when we respect each other's customs and traditions, recognize that the end of December means different things to different people, and find joy in learning about new ways of celebrating.

And that's the perspective Ellen brings to the world, not just with this book, but with her entire body of work. Ellen and I share a love of the seasonal festivals and a fascination with their customs and enactments worldwide. She has been writing books about the diversity of Pagan traditions for many years, offering a wealth of information for anyone with an interest in herbs, plant magic, and folklore. *The Sacred Herbs of Yule and Christmas* is now my favorite. I hope you enjoy reading it as much as I have. I hope it becomes a beloved reference of wintertime recipes and folklore for you to delve into in all the years to come.

Lucya Starza is the author of *Scrying, Candle Magic, Guided Visualisations,* and *Poppets and Magical Dolls* in the Pagan Portals series. She edited the community book *Every Day Magic* and is the author of *A Bad Witch's Blog,* a blog about Paganism, Witchcraft, and the day-to-day experiences of a London Witch, which can be found at **www.badwitch.co.uk**. She is a Gardnerian Wiccan and lives in London with her husband and cats.

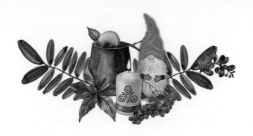

An Introduction to Yule and Herbal Magic

In the bleak midwinter, frosty wind made moan,
Earth stood hard as iron, water like a stone;
Snow had fallen, snow on snow, snow on snow,
In the bleak midwinter, long ago.

Christina Rossetti,
"In the Bleak Midwinter" (1872)

As chill winds bear down, nature fades from her autumnal greens and amber to the steely whites and gray of the snowbound landscape. Nights grow ever darker, but the denuded trees offer no barrier to the vault of the heavens, letting in ever more starlight. The Moon is in Her glory, too, unimpeded by obscuring branches. Orion the Hunter is on the rise, and the Pleiades dance.

As if to combat the growing cold and longer nights, right on cue, the colors red, white, green, and gold appear everywhere, assaulting our senses. In any other season those colors would seem harsh, garish, clashing wildly, yet at this time of year they feel just right. They seem to offer comfort and cheer to tide us across the yawning abyss of the blackest season, which, in the not-so-distant past, might have brought starvation, sickness, and want.

Red is the color of blood and of fire, and by extension of the Sun and of lightning. These are the forces that embody warmth, power, energy, and protection. Red symbolizes the "good red road" of Lakota tradition, meaning a life guided by sacred precepts and virtues—spirituality, living rightly, wisdom.[1]

White is the color of snow, of course, but it also symbolizes cleanliness and purity, faith, righteousness, and peace.[2] White is also associated with death; in Slavic traditions, it implies the thin veil between the living and the dead, between Earth and sky, between death and rebirth, a fitting reminder of the snows of winter under which the vegetation slumbers in apparent demise before the plants spring to green life once more.[3]

Green is the color of life, carried through the dead of winter by evergreen trees that reveal their full glory only once deciduous leaves have dropped and decayed. Their scent and vibrant color remind us that life carries on, even in the darkest cold of winter.

Gold is the color of stars, glowing through naked branches on a winter's night. In mystical traditions, gold is symbolic of the Alpha and the Omega, the Source and End of all things—a fitting emblem of the dying year and its eventual rebirth.

Ancient Origins of the Yule Festival

Yule is the word for the ancient northern European winter festival that spans the Solstice season. The original Yule celebrations lasted from mid-November to mid-January, comprising great festivals and invocations of light and fire, spanning the coldest, darkest season. This was also the time when farm animals were slaughtered, so there was plenty of meat for feasting—and a lot of alcohol consumption.

Danish Vikings brought Yule to Britain in the ninth and tenth centuries, and by the thirteenth century it had become attached to Christmas ceremonies. But the traditional Christian celebration of Jesus's birth on December 25 itself arises from more ancient, pre-Christian roots. It was Mithras, the Persian God of light, of the rising Sun, of contracts, covenants, and friendship, the all-seeing protector of truth, and the guardian of cattle, the harvest, and the waters, who was originally said to have been born on December 25.

Mithras was popular with Roman soldiers, and by the fourth century he was linked to Sol Invictus (Unconquered Sun) as the official Sun God of the Roman Empire. Roman Christians eventually adopted Mithras's date of birth and powerful all-seeing solar attributes, grafting them onto their savior Jesus of Nazareth.[4]

As you'll read throughout this book, many of our modern traditions arise from ancient roots. Our modern Santa Claus may be a secular version of Saint Nicholas, a fourth-century bishop who liked to distribute aid to the needy. Or he may be a modern version of Odin or Neptune, both bearded men who traveled widely and protected sailors. Others say he is the incarnation of a shamanic mushroom Spirit, seen by Siberian shamans when they partake of *Amanita muscaria*—a red mushroom with white spots that is still a feature of Christmas decorations in Scandinavia and other northern areas.

Four thousand years ago, the ancient Egyptians decorated their homes with greenery, such as the fronds of the date palm, at the festival celebrating the rebirth of the God Horus (the son of the Goddess Isis who was born hanging in a tree). The festival was a twelve-day observance in honor of the returning Sun and also a celebration of the completion of the date harvest.

Meanwhile, the ancient Romans decorated their homes with vines and other greenery and shared gifts, especially candles, at the midwinter festival of Saturnalia, in honor of the agricultural God and lord of the harvest, Saturn. They hung metal ornaments on trees, usually depictions of Saturn or the deity of the household, and celebrated with feasting, merrymaking, drinking, gambling, wandering the streets naked, singing songs, and generally making as much mischief as possible.

In Scandinavian and Germanic areas in midwinter, families burned a Yule Log in the hearth, wassailed their fruit orchards, and displayed sheaves of Wheat, because if you were lucky enough to have a good Wheat harvest, your display of it carried the luck into the new year. Germanic tribes decorated trees with fruits and candles in Odin's honor at the Solstice.

In Celtic areas, mummers and guisers went from home to home spreading the Spirit of the Land Goddess throughout the villages, and Druids gathered Mistletoe as a medicinal and magical aid.

All of these traditions (and many, many more) have come down to us with a certain mix-and-match character. We erect Christmas trees and decorate them with ornaments and lights. We string lights outside our homes, hang Mistletoe and Holly, and go caroling with neighbors or at church. We honor the birth of a God, invoke the powers of Spirits to protect us from the dark, and stand in ritual to ask the Sun to return. We visit, gift, toast, dance, feast, and drink a-plenty.

Some of us faithfully practice time-honored family, cultural, or religious rituals. Others simply enjoy the merrymaking. Still others gather to honor the turn of the Wheel of the Year. Regardless of our particular tradition or inclination, the time of the Winter Solstice, Yule, Christmas, and New Year's is filled with meaning and magic. This book explores the roots of this ancient celebration from the magical and medicinal herbs of winter to the traditions, rites, foods, and drinks of the season, with the intention of deepening our understanding of the past so that we can carry it forward with purpose, respect, and joy.

Herbal Magic

In all my books, I include both the magical uses of herbs and their herbal healing properties. I am careful to separate the two because they are different ways of seeing and working with plants, yet both approaches are valid. One is more physical, while the other addresses the mental and emotional concerns that often accompany an illness or other life crisis.

Plants have many spheres of action. There are herbal brews, homeopathic dilutions, flower essences, oils, poultices and salves, incenses and magical potions, each of which resonates with a different stratum of the body, psyche, and spirit. Among all of these octaves of the healer's art, one thing is common: Plants *want* to heal us.

Plants are a physical manifestation of the love of the Earth. If we pay attention, we notice that the very plants we need will pop up in our gardens or even on the city block where we regularly walk. Mother Nature is always trying to heal and feed her children. I vividly remember the year 2008, when everyone was in a panic over the stock market crash caused by reckless American banks and mortgage companies. Many of us (including me) lost savings, while others were driven to despair. Some of us had no idea how to cover the cost of basics such as rent and food, and many people lost their homes.

That was a mast year for the Oaks in my area. I remember walking outside and it was raining Acorns—literally manna from heaven. I took full advantage and made an extra-large portion of Acorn flour, which I used for breads and cakes all winter. The same thing happened in 2021, in the midst of the SARS Covid-19 epidemic, when people were afraid to leave their homes, go to a job, or be in a public area. Once again, the manna came raining down. The pity is that so few people know how to use these gifts from our common parent, Mother Earth.

Plants have Spirits that we can communicate with when we show them gratitude and respect. They are sentient beings and allies. When we tune in to the natural world—to the plants, animals, waters, winds, Sun, Moon, Earth—we begin to see that these beings, entities, and forces surround us, support us, and call to us. We ignore them at our own peril.

As a species, we need to learn to contain ourselves, to find the humility of our reliance on the rest of the natural world, to find the joy and awe of participation in a web of interconnectedness that defies our capacity to grasp. We need to stop assaulting nature. We need to be mindful of where we choose to build and how we use natural resources. Behind and beyond all the artifice of cultivation and construction, the natural world is our home. We need the wild to stay wild.

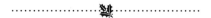

I wish to acknowledge the contributions of my amazing editor Meghan MacLean. Many thanks to Kevin Sartoris whose opinions always help to shape my books. And my deep gratitude to Lucya Starza for the lovely foreword.

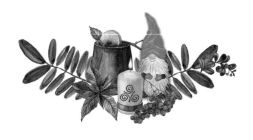

A Primer on Herbal Preparation

Before we foray into the Yuletide herbs that heal us, protect us, and help us contact the Spirits, let's talk about the different methods of finding and preparing herbs.

Finding Good-Quality Herbs

You can grow herbs yourself, purchase them from commercial growers, or wild-craft—that is, collect them from the wild. However, there are some considerations to take into account.

First, before you head into the wild to gather plants, make sure of their status in your area. A number of the plants listed in this book are now threatened or endangered due to overharvesting and habitat loss. Keep the following rule in mind: "Walk by the first seven, leave the eighth for the animals, and you may take the ninth." This practice ensures conservation; there will be enough plants left in the wild to produce seed for the following year, and the creatures of the wild will have the food they depend on.

Because overharvesting of wild populations is such a problem, do not purchase wild-crafted herbs unless you know they are of a species that is very abundant. Instead, purchase commercially grown herbs. Be sure that these herbs are organic, because nonorganic commercially grown herbs tend to be heavily contaminated with pesticides. This is especially true for plants that come from other countries (China, India); imported plants may also be irradiated.

How to Make a Tea

Herbal teas can generally be divided into two categories—infusions and decoctions—depending on which part of the plant is being brewed. The rule of thumb is that flowers and leaves, being more delicate plant parts, are prepared as infusions, while the tougher plant parts, like roots, barks, and seeds, are prepared as decoctions.

Infusion: Bring water to a boil, pour the hot water over the herbs, cover, and let steep for about 20 minutes.

Decoction: Combine the water and herbs in a nonaluminum pot, cover tightly, bring to a simmer, and let simmer for about 20 minutes. (Never boil your herbs; they will lose their volatile oils through the steam.)

Whether you're making an infusion or a decoction, the usual proportions are 2 teaspoons of herbs per cup of water (use a bit more if the herbs are fresh—about 2½ teaspoons). The dose is ¼ cup taken four times a day, not with meals. The idea is to have a small amount of the herb in your system all day.

How to Make a Salve

Put your fresh, wilted, or dry herbs in a nonaluminum pot and add just enough cold-pressed virgin oil (Olive oil is the best one for general purposes) to barely cover them. Keep careful track of how much oil you pour into the pot.

Cover the pot, bring the oil to a simmer, and let simmer (do not boil) for at least 20 minutes. Or bring to a simmer and then turn off the heat, repeating that process several times a day for a week, allowing the herbs to steep continuously in the hot oil.

In a separate pot, bring beeswax to the same temperature as the simmering hot oil. Put 3 to 4 tablespoons of hot beeswax per cup of oil used into the pot with the herbs. Stir well and then strain the hot mixture into very clean glass jars or metal tins. Cap tightly and store in a cool, dark place.

How to Make a Poultice

Put fresh herbs into a blender (or pour boiling hot water over dried herbs to make them soft and then put them in the blender). Add just enough water so that you can blend the herbs into a "mush."

Pour the mush into a bowl and mix in just enough powdered Slippery Elm (*Ulmus rubra*) bark for the mixture to take on the consistency of pie dough. In a pinch you can use Buckwheat flour, potato flour or mashed potato, or rice flour (avoid Wheat flour, because some people are allergic to Wheat) or omit the thickener altogether and simply spread the blended or softened herbs onto a cloth and apply to the area. However, Slippery Elm is loaded with calcium and it will speed skin and bone healing, which is why I usually add it to my poultices.

Lightly knead the mixture into a ball.

Set the ball on a clean cloth. Use a rolling pin or an old bottle to roll it out flat. Apply the poultice to the body, laying the flattened herb mixture directly on the skin and wrapping the cloth as needed to hold it in place. Keep the poultice on for 1 hour, then remove it and discard the herb mixture.

Poultices are best applied cold, so try making them ahead of time and freezing them or storing them in the refrigerator before use.

How to Make a Fomentation

A fomentation is like a hot, moist poultice. First, steam or simmer the herbs in a very minimal amount of water until soft. Soak a very clean cloth in the herbal brew and then lay out the hot cloth on a plate. Transfer the cooked herbs to the cloth and fold it to keep the herbs inside. Apply to the body while still warm.

How to Make a Tincture

Pack your herbs into a glass jar and add just enough vodka to barely cover them. (Plain vodka is best, although anything that is at least 80 percent alcohol, such as whiskey, will do in a pinch.) Cap tightly and let steep, shaking the jar periodically (at least a few times a week).

Pay careful attention to your herbs. When the plant matter begins to break down—this can take a just few hours for flowers, a few days for leaves, and a few weeks for roots, barks, berries, or fungi—strain out the liquid. Store the tincture in a dark place or in a blue or brown glass bottle. Be sure to put a label and a date on the bottle so you remember what it is!

Adding a few drops of vegetable glycerin to the "mother tincture" (I use about 1 teaspoon per quart) will make the tincture more bioavailable. Vegetable glycerin increases the valency of the herb's molecules, meaning that each molecule will have more electrons sticking out of it so that the body's receptors will have an easier time latching on.

The usual dose for tinctures is 20 drops, taken in hot tea or water, three or four times a day. That dose assumes a 150-pound person. Someone who weighs significantly more or less should adjust the dose accordingly; for example, a 75-pound person would get half the usual dose. Nursing mothers with a sick infant can take the tincture in hot water or tea, which will pass the effects on to their baby.

A number of edible herbs, including Cayenne, Lobelia, Nettles, Dandelion, Violet flower, Chive blossom, and Red Clover, are best tinctured in vinegar rather than vodka. Vinegar tinctures are helpful for children and for people who wish to avoid alcohol. Vinegar tinctures last about 2 years, while alcohol tinctures last about 5 years.

Using Essential Oils

Essential oils are the volatile aromatic oils found in plant material. They are potent! They can be used externally or for aromatherapeutic applications. Irritation or allergic reaction could occur when applying essential oils to the skin, so practice care: Do a skin patch test before using any new essential oil, and never apply to the skin undiluted. Pregnant or nursing women and children should consult their health-care providers before using any essential oil.

Essential oils should be stored in a dark brown or blue bottle and kept in a cool, dark place.

Cautions

Many herbs should be avoided by people with a number of medical conditions, like diabetes or high blood pressure, and by people who are taking certain medications, whether over-the-counter or prescription. So, if you have any serious health problems or are taking any medication and you want to try using a particular herb, please check the contraindications for that herb. You can search online for "herb-drug interaction" or use the Natural Medicines Comprehensive Database. WebMD often has good advice too, and an herbalist or naturopath will be able to give you good guidance as well.

The same holds true if you are pregnant or breastfeeding—check for contraindications before beginning to use an herb. Some herbs can lead to complications in pregnancy, while others are unsafe for infants and can be passed through to them via the mother's breast milk.

As is the case with most foods and medicines, herbs that are perfectly safe for most people can stimulate a bad reaction in certain individuals. So, if you have never used a particular herb, before diving in, first try a small amount and see how it affects you.

Above all, if I say something is poisonous, I mean it! If an herb is especially dangerous but you'd still like to use it, you can safely partake of it via a homeopathic dilution or flower essence.

If you are healthy, if you are not taking medications, and if you pay careful attention to the cautions associated with each plant, you should be able to work with the herbs as described in the following chapters. Alternatively, you can simply place them on your altar or wear them on your person as a crown or in an amulet bag, charm bag, mojo bag, or medicine bundle.

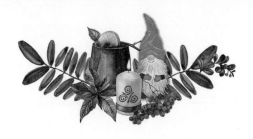

A Primer on Herb Magic

Hedge Witchery and Hedge Druidry involve working with what you find around you, and that includes plants. Any plant you are attracted to can be partnered with to manifest what you need if you follow a few basic principles.

First and foremost, **ask permission**! First ground and center. Slow your breathing as you approach the plant and see if it *wants* to give of itself. Touch it with your hand, use a pendulum, or try other methods of questioning. If you get a "yes," you may proceed.

Magical Properties of Plants

Below are descriptions of some of the magical properties of plants to aid in your partnering.

Magical Properties of Plant Parts

Roots: Roots are to help you ground. They are familiar with the Underworld of the Sidhe (Fairies), the beloved dead, and Underworld deities. Wear roots, eat them, or drink their tea when you seek grounding, want to contact the ancestors, or want to understand hidden forces and dark secrets.

Bark: The outer bark of trees and shrubs is protective. Wear the bark or drink a bark tea to strengthen your personal shields.

Leaves: Leaves are manifestations of energy and growth. Drink leaf teas, eat leaves, and wear them to increase your strength, enthusiasm, and will to keep going.

Highly Aromatic Plants: Aromatic herbs and resins have disinfectant properties. Use these plants for healing, purification, and the consecration of persons, places, and things.

Flowers: Flowers are the sex organs of plants. Use their fragrance and beauty to increase your personal magnetism and attractiveness and for greater fertility and sexual pleasure. Drink a flower tea or add flowers to your bath to lighten your spirit and attract love.

Fruits: Fruits are the ultimate manifestation of a plant's life work. Fruits are all about wealth, abundance, and success. Eat fruits to both cleanse and build your body.

Nuts and Seeds: Every seed holds within it the potential for a new beginning. Seeds contain the possibilities of transition, change, renewal of cycles, and the future. Seeds such as Walnuts ease mental struggles and nourish the brain.

Magical Properties of the Color of Plants

Yellow flowers are Solar and impart courage, generosity, and will power.

Red flowers, fruits, and berries bring passion and vitality.

Pink flowers denote love and tender emotion.

White flowers imply spiritual love for all beings and sometimes death.

Blue flowers are a sign of optimism and altruism.

Purple flowers are keys to magic and the mysteries.

Orange flowers mean health for the whole body.

Green flowers and leaves bring balance and peace.

Black flowers and berries are very deeply connected to the astral world and can protect you from malignant forces.

Seasonal Magic of Plants

Spring Gathering: Spring is the time when the sap is rising. Spring gathered plants, especially those picked during the Waxing Moon, bring energy to new projects and relationships. Plants gathered on the eve of the Beltaine Full Moon are the most potent of all.

Summer Gathering: The time of Summer Solstice when the Sun is at its height is the most auspicious time to gather above ground plants for medicine. Magically, these herbs help with manifestation and with dissolving blockages.

Fall Gathering: Fall gathered roots act deeply with long-lasting effects. They help to understand the mysteries and to make contact with the Underworld of the Faeries and the Ancestors.

Winter Gathering: Plants that stay green all winter are very wise. They are the ultimate survivors, bestowing practical solutions and clarity, strength, endurance, grit, persistence, and long life. Plants that thrive in the baking heat and freezing cold of arid deserts have similar qualities.

Crafting Spells

Spells do not have a time limit or constraint; they can manifest quickly or may take years. A large intention can take a decade of visualization, while a smaller working could happen almost instantly.

In this book, I have included a few chants to sing or recite as you make your herbal brews. Practice crafting your own! As you chant, visualize the outcome you desire. Hold the faith that it will happen, in its own time. Don't worry about exact timing—just "be still and know."

Visualize the outcome as *already happening*. If you or someone you know is sick, see them as fully healed. If someone is depressed, visualize them as joyful and productive. Project colors as needed: pink for love, red for passion, orange for vitality, yellow for intellect and courage, green for balance, blue for peace, purple for magic and the mysteries, black for protection. Decorate your altar and choose flowers and fruits for magic based on their colors.

Make your thoughts as clear and focused as possible. Consciousness is everywhere and in all things. The universe will pick up on your desire if you send out a clear intention.

Basic Steps to Creative Spell Work

Grounding: Connect with the Earth below your feet. Visualize yourself as a tree or plant, with roots going deep into the ground. *See* your roots going all the way down to the center of the Earth, the green, luminous heart of our Mother.

Cleaning House: Clean the house from top to bottom. Don't forget the kitchen and bathroom (or even the windows!). Sweep out old energies, and leave a door or window cracked open so the nasties can escape. Wash the floors with a purifying herbal blend. Take a shower and allow the water to cleanse your chakras, rinsing any blockages down the drain.

Shielding: Select a protective herb and wear it on your person. Visualize a ring of protection, of white light, like a glowing hoop around your body; a protective force field that repels all negativity.

The Altar: Cleanse and refresh your altar. Wash the altar cloth. Set up fresh herbs and flowers as appropriate to the work. Set out fresh new candles, and clean any crystals, statues, and stones. Your robes, too, should be clean and fresh.

Drink a Potion: Make an herbal potion based on the properties I have described in this book. (See also my books *The Sacred Herbs of Spring* and *The Sacred Herbs of Samhain* for more seasonal potions.)

Cleansing with Smoke: Burn herbs as incense (or make an herbal spray if you are sensitive to the smoke). Use the smoke (or liquid) to purify the ritual area, ritual tools, and celebrants.

Make a Libation: Pour a brew onto the ground as an offering for Underworld entities and Spirits.

Offerings to Fire: Offer dried herbs, oil, ghee, or alcohol (or other things that fire likes) to the fire. Place fragrant herbs in the fire as an offering to the sky world of the deities, or burn incense in their honor.

Open a Portal between the Worlds: Ask the Spirits to open the veil so that deities and magical helpers may travel to you freely.

Call on the Gods and Goddesses: Now you are ready to call on the deities you work with. Petition them for help and then ask them what they require from you in exchange.

Divine the Outcome: Do a divination to be sure you understand what the Goddesses and Gods require of you and to find out whether your petition was accepted (and if it wasn't, start over).

Closing the Portal: Give thanks to all the Spirits and entities you petitioned for aid. Ask that the portal between the worlds be closed and that only the good remain.

Retract Your Roots: Unwind your roots from the luminous green heart of Earth and from the soil beneath your feet. Visualize yourself as fully human again. *Know* that all shall be well!

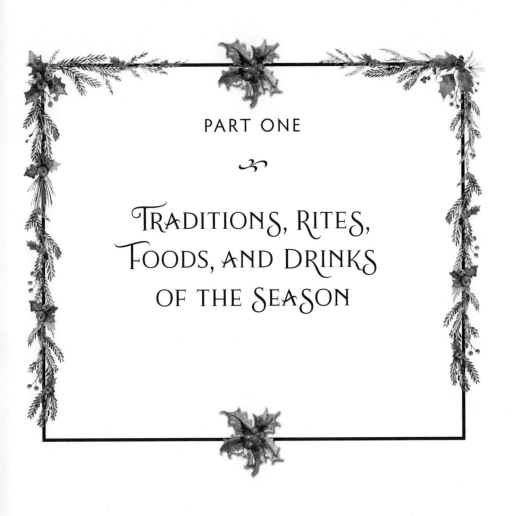

PART ONE

જી

Traditions, Rites, Foods, and Drinks of the Season

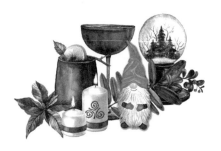

The Gift Bringers, Spirits, and Mystical Figures of Winter

Benign gift bringers are part of cultural lore in many areas. Generosity is reinforced by the stories and traditions of gift sharing in the harsh season of winter—the idea of distributing food and valuables among relatives, children, and even the poor is an ancient expression of the willingness to help one's family and community survive the winter. Frightening gift bringers (and withholders) appear as well to remind us to behave or we won't be rewarded and of the ever-present danger and ferocity that lurk behind the beauty of winter's cold and snow.

Santa Claus and Other Gift Bringers

Families and communities have been sharing gifts during the winter season for millennia. In modern times a male figure known as Father Christmas, Santa Claus, or Saint Nick has become popular, but in ancient times female gift bringers and Spirits were anticipated at Yule. Here we'll explore this range of gift bringers both ancient and modern.

Saint Nicholas

Saint Nicholas was a fourth-century bishop who was born in Turkey, imprisoned by the emperor Diocletian, and set free by Constantine and attended the First Council of Nicaea in the year 325 CE. Legend has it that he gave gold to a poor man's daughters to save them from prostitution and brought three murdered boys back to life. Through these acts, he became associated with children and with generosity. After he died, he became the patron saint of Russia and Greece, as well as choir boys, thieves, perfumers, barrel makers, single women, and sailors.

The remains of Saint Nicholas were taken from an Orthodox church in Myra, Turkey, and secreted away to Bari, Italy, where his grave is said to exude a sweet-smelling manna. His feast day is December 6, and by the year 1100 it became practice to give presents to children (or at least children from noble families) on that day. Eventually, nuns in Italy started leaving out presents for poor children, and in 1531 Martin Luther instructed German children to leave out their stockings to be filled. English children waited by the window for him to come in, bearing gifts. The Protestant Reformation saw his eventual replacement by the Christ Child, and gift giving was moved to December 25 or to New Year's Day. In 1969 the Catholic church demoted Saint Nicholas to a minor saint who is only optionally venerated.[1]

In the nineteenth century, Santa Claus, whose name and attributes descend directly from those of Saint Nicholas, became a fabled gift bringer in the lore of the United States. He is said to visit each home by coming down the chimney (even when we don't have a chimney!). He is dressed in red and white, colors that some associate with the red and white Fly Agaric or Amanita mushroom (*Amanita muscaria*) that is eaten by reindeer and shamans in the polar areas that Santa Claus is said to hail from. Others opine that his reindeer-drawn sleigh is somehow related to the Scandinavian God Odin's eight-legged horse Sleipnir, which he rides across the sky.

Children leave out food for Santa and his reindeer—cookies, milk, and a carrot or two—a practice that may be related to the old European belief in extending hospitality toward the wandering dead and the ancestors on high holy days (similarly, an extra place may be set at the table for any dead ancestors who happen by).

Santa's Scary Helpers

In the Netherlands, Saint Nicholas is often accompanied by his "helper," Zwarte Piet (Black Peter), who flings candy at good children and threatens to abduct bad ones. Black Peter is a controversial figure in Holland these days. His origins are no older than the mid 1800s, a time when the Dutch were engaged in colonialism and the slave trade. Some now perceive him as nothing more than a demonized caricature of a black man, while others claim he is just sooty because he came down the chimney.[2]

In Austria, he is accompanied by Klaubauf, a scary figure with dark, shaggy fur and the horns of a goat, dressed in rags and clanking chains. In lower Austria, it is Krampus who comes with the saint, looking like a horned Demon carrying a whip. He has a basket on his back in which to capture bad children. When Krampus threatens someone (for example, in a public parade), though, Saint Nicholas always steps in to intercede.

In some parts of Germany, Saint Nicholas has a helper called Belsnickel or Pelznickel (from *pelzen* or *belzen,* German for "to wallop" or "to drub"), who questions kids to see if they have been bad or good. He carries a switch and wears a cap, a fur cape, bells, and a chain. In other German traditions, the Schimmelreiter (Ghost Rider), a bogeyman along the lines of Krampus, is said to accompany Saint Nicholas.[3]

Mrs. Claus

Mrs. Claus is a well-known modern purveyor of gifts—she helps her husband, Santa, in his yearly work of gift manufacturing and distribution, though depictions of her usually have her staying at home at the North Pole, baking cookies, on delivery day. Like Santa, she is an international figure with different aliases in various languages: Mother Christmas (English), Weihnachtsfrau, (German), Joulumuori (Finnish), Bayan Noel (Turkish), and La Mère Noël (French).

Mrs. Claus travels with Saint Nicholas on occasion; she is known as Niglofrau (Nicholas's wife) in Austria, Nicolaaswijf in Holland, and Nikoloweibl in Bavaria. In the Austrian Tirol, Klasa (the feminine form of Claus) sometimes travels with the saint, handing out presents from a basket.

Other Gift Bringers

In Romania, children put out their shoes in hopes that they will be filled with candy and gifts on December 5, the eve of Saint Nicholas's day. But naughty children will find only a switch. The Romanian version of Santa, Moş Crăciun (Old Father Christmas), comes down the chimney on Christmas Eve.

In the Basque area that straddles northeastern Spain and southwestern France, a character called Olentzero (whose name means "time of the good ones"), originally a giant and later described as a charcoal burner or shepherd, comes down from the wild mountains on the night of December 24 to distribute presents. He wears a *boina*, a Basque beret. On Christmas Eve, Basque shepherds dance in the village, wearing pelts and reciting ancient verses.[4] Youths go from house to house, dancing and singing, collecting food or money to prepare a festive dinner.

The Swedish Jultomte, Norwegian Julenisse, Danish Julemand, and Finnish Joulupukki (each name translates roughly to "Christmas Elf") is a Spirit, Gnome, or Pixie-like character that helps with chores in the house and on the farm. These beings may groom horses, carry bales of hay, and help with other farmyard tasks, which they do more efficiently than humans, so long as they are bribed with food (like a nice bowl of porridge with a pat of butter). In most stories, they are described as temperamental, red-capped, and short (under 4 feet tall), and feature most commonly in the lore of Denmark, southern Norway, and southern Sweden. At Christmas time, they bring gifts for their households. Rather than coming down the chimney, they come right in through the front door.

In some parts of Sweden, the Julbukk (Yule buck or Christmas goat) brings gifts, pulling a Jultomte with a red cap and long white beard. This story echoes the mythology of ancient Pagan Scandinavia in which two goats pulled the God Thor across the sky, adding a mystical dimension to the Christmas Goat.[5]

In Russia, Ded Moroz (Grandfather Frost)—the official Soviet replacement figure for Saint Nicholas—is the gift bringer. His helper, Snegurochka (Snow Maiden), appears only in winter, presiding over the New Year's festivities. She retreats to the north in summer. She is said to have long blond hair and wears a blue-and-white fur-lined costume. Other Russian traditions speak of Babushka, the cranky "Old Woman" who refused to visit the newborn Jesus. Some accounts tell that she even gave the Magi wrong directions on purpose! On the eve of Epiphany (January 6), she is said to bring presents to sleeping children.[6]

In Czech areas, on December 4, the eve of Saint Barbara's Day, women dress as the Barborky (Barbaras), in white dresses and veils, carrying baskets of sweets for good children and brooms to threaten the naughty. On December 8, the day of the Feast of the Immaculate Conception, Matíčka (the Blessed Mother) might leave treats in children's shoes.[7]

In France, from the Middle Ages into the nineteenth century, people left out food and drink at night for Lady Abundia, Domine Habundie, or Satia, the gift bringer of New Year's. She was a later version of Abundantia, the ancient Roman Goddess of prosperity and abundance whose name literally means "plenty" or "overflowing riches" and who brought good luck and fortune to those she visited.[8]

The French also have La Tante Airie, a kind fairy who is said to be the reincarnation of the medieval French countess Henriette de Montbéliard. La Tante Airie takes people who have been frozen by the cold into her grotto and miraculously warms their hearts once more. Always accompanied by her donkey, she listens to children's wishes, which are carried to her by the wind. She leaves nice presents for good children, while leaving the naughty ones nothing but a boot full of twigs.

In Italy, La Befana, the Christmas Witch, is the bringer of presents. According to legend, she was invited to join the Magi on their journey to visit the newborn Christ Child but preferred to stay at home and clean house. She seems to have regretted that decision because she now wanders the world seeking the child, dropping down chimneys and leaving gifts for good children but only ashes for those who misbehave. She very sensibly wears black because it doesn't show the soot![9]

Mother Goody, who originated in Scotland, is the spirit of New Year's in New Brunswick, Canada. Children hang their stockings on New Year's Eve for her to fill. Aunt Nancy or Mother New Year also brings New Year's gifts in Canada; children hang their stockings in hopes that she will fill them. In some Canadian areas, "Queen Mab," the Christmas Fairy, puts gifts into stockings on Christmas Eve—but naughty children find only a birch rod.[10]

Similarly, Hertha, the Norse Goddess of the hearth, is said to grace the household fire at midwinter. She comes down the chimney bringing the gift of good luck to the household. Her presence in the fireplace may be one of the origins of the pervasive concept of Christmas gift bringers coming down the chimney.[11] A related German Yuletide figure called Lutzelfrau, said to ride the wind at midwinter, brings gifts such as apples, nuts, and dried plums to children on Saint Lucy's Day (December 13).[12]

In Poland, presents are brought by Gwiazdor (whose name means "Star Man" or "Man from the Stars"), who was originally a western Slavic winter deity who delivered gifts at the Winter Solstice. He is typically dressed in a fur or woven straw coat and wears a wooden mask with a straw beard attached. He has a high cap of woven straw, leather, or fur and carries birch rods to threaten children who have been naughty. Gwiazdor may be accompanied by Gwiazdka (whose name means "Little Star" or "Star Woman"), who is sometimes called Piękna Pani (meaning "Beautiful Lady"). Gwiazdka is a silent companion to Gwiazdor. She wears a long white dress, a veil, and a crown of flowers and greenery with straw and ribbons woven through it. (These deified star references are in honor of the Sun. Before Christianity, the Slavic people celebrated the Winter Solstice as the feast of the reborn Sun.)[13]

Other Yule season gift bringers are legion. Father Christmas brings presents in British areas, Père Noël in French-speaking regions, and Baba Noel in the Middle East. Among some devout Catholics, it is Baby Jesus (or El Niño in some Latin American cultures) who makes gifts appear. In Spain, the Three Kings drop off gifts on January 5, on their way to Bethlehem. In Syria, the Magi's youngest camel brings the presents, while in Lebanon, it's a mule.[14]

In Alsace, La Dame de Noel (the Lady of Christmas) brings gifts.[15] In the Cantabrian Mountains, Fairies known as *anjanas* bring gifts every four years on January 6. In the Dominican Republic, La Vieja

Belén (The Old Lady of Bethlehem) brings presents to poor children on January 6. In Switzerland, on Christmas Eve a girl dressed in white carries a lantern through the town, representing the Christ Child. A retinue of six other girls accompanies her, singing carols and distributing gifts.[16]

Demons, Trolls, Elves, and Other Fearsome Spirits

Grýla and the Yule Lads

In Iceland, December 12 is the time to begin rituals to repel evil Spirits with bright lights, noise, and incense. Two mystical figures who are likely to show up in the streets are the Trolls Grýla and her husband, Leppalúði, who are fond of eating naughty children (and sometimes fully grown men), whom they capture in their sack and then boil in a huge cauldron. According to the Icelandic Sturlunga saga, compiled sometime around the year 1300, Grýla has fifteen tails and three hundred heads, with three eyes on each head. The nails on her fingers are rotten. She has horns like a goat. Her ears dangle down to her shoulders and are fastened to her nose, while her chin is bearded and her teeth are black as charcoal.

According to Icelandic lore, Grýla's pet, known as the Christmas Cat, will eat anyone who does not get at least one item of new clothing at Christmas. This story, it's thought, originates from the tradition of giving the spinners and knitters who had labored all year a reward of clothing for their hard work.[17]

Among Grýla and Leppalúði's children are the thirteen Yule Lads, who come to town, one by one, each night from December 12 to December 24. The Lads are ugly, boorish louts who dress in peasant costumes from ancient times. They are reputedly cannibalistic, just like their mom and dad, with names that fit their personalities: Stekkjastaur (Sheep Cote Clod), who likes to harass the sheep; Giljagaur (Gully Gawk), who breaks into the barn to steal milk; Stufur (Stubby), who is short and likes to steal pots and pans; Thvorusleikir (Spoon Licker), who likes to lick off any food left on dirty spoons; Pottaskefill (Pot Scraper), who breaks into the house and steals any leftover food; Askasleikir (Bowl Licker), a monster who hides under children's beds and emerges at night to slurp the remains of whatever is left in bowls; Hurdaskellir (Door Slammer), who roams from house to house and breaks in to slam and bang as many doors as he can; Skyrgamur (Skyr Gobbler), who lusts after skyr, the Icelandic version of yogurt; Bjugnakraekir (Sausage Snatcher), who hides in the rafters and swoops down to steal sausages being smoked; Gluggagaegir (Window Peeper), who spies on children through windows at night; Gattathefur (Doorway Sniffer), who has a huge nose and is always sniffing around doorways looking for his favorite food, Icelandic *laufabrauð* (leaf bread); Ketkrókur (Meat Hook), who hides in the kitchen and uses a hook to steal meat; and Kertasnikir (Candle Stealer), who steals candles from children so they can't read in the dark (reading is a favorite Icelandic activity, especially on long winter nights).

After thirteen days of mischief and rampage, the thirteen Lads, their parents Grýla and Leppalúði, and the Christmas Cat all retreat to the far distant mountains, where they remain until the next Yule.[18]

The Kallikantzari

The Greek Kallikantzari are Elves or Demons who are said to appear during the twelve-day period between Christmas and Epiphany (January 6). Descriptions of their appearance vary. They are said to be small, black, male, and mostly blind, with long black tails, or perhaps to have crooked legs and arms, hunched backs, large ears, strange eyes, and all kinds of other deformities. Some report that they wear wooden or iron boots to better kick people; others maintain that they are hooved, not booted. Their speech is lisping, and they like to dine on worms, snails, and frogs.

The Kallikantzari live deep underground at the center of the Earth, where they constantly labor with a huge handsaw to cut down the World Tree that supports the Earth. They are terrified of the Sun and emerge only at Yuletide, during the darkest days of the year. Once aboveground, they invade homes, coming down the chimney and through openings such as keyholes, windows, and cracks in doors and windows. They play tricks on humans, perhaps peeing on the fire, souring the milk, or making people dance to the point of exhaustion, and generally cause mayhem.

The best way to control them is by fire, which they are deathly afraid of. For this reason, a large Yule Log is kept burning in the hearth for the entire Yuletide period. You can also repel them by hanging herbs of protection and purification, such as Hyssop, Thistle, and Asparagus, or the jaw of a pig. You can leave a kitchen colander on the doorstep to distract them, because they are so stupid that they can only count to two and will get lost counting the holes in the colander all night.

The Kallikantzari retreat after Epiphany, and their departure can be hastened by sprinkling the house with blessed water using a sprig of fresh Basil. Upon their return to their underground home, they find that the World Tree has magically regenerated, which infuriates them, and they begin attacking it all over again.[19]

Werewolves

Another troublesome Yuletide Spirit is the Werewolf. Olaus Magnus, a Swedish ecclesiastic and historian writing in the Middle Ages, reported that in Lithuania, Livonia, and Poland, Werewolves roamed on Christmas Eve to "rage with wonderous ferocity" against humans. They would try to break down doors and, if successful, devour any person or animal they could find. They would also play monster games with each other, and the loser was eaten!

In Latvia and Estonia, stories tell of an innocent-looking little lame boy who wanders the countryside summoning Satan's followers to a gathering. Anyone who lags behind is beaten with an iron whip. In the end, they all transform into wolves and remain in that form for the twelve days of Christmas.

In Poland and northeastern Europe, it was once said that any child born on Christmas had a greater chance of becoming a Werewolf.

In one tradition rooted in the swampy regions of Louisiana, Père Noël (Father Christmas) is said to cross the bayous at night in a boat pulled by alligators and a red-nosed Werewolf.[20]

Other Frightful Figures

Sometimes Yuletide Spirits roam the Earth in broad daylight, walking right through the middle of town. In Austria, the Perchtenlaufen folk tradition, taking place in December, is ritual pageantry, symbolic of the battle between winter and spring, darkness and light, civilization and wild nature, goodness and evil. The hairy, horned Spirit called Krampus stalks the streets, making loud noises with bells and drums while, simultaneously, beautiful figures mysteriously appear in the roadways and squares.

In Czech regions, a black-clad Čert (Devil), travels with an Anděl (Angel) dressed in white alongside Saint Mikulas (Nicholas). They arrive on the evening of December 5. The Čert shows up carrying a sack, a whip, and a chain to terrify badly behaved boys and girls. Each child recites a poem or sings a song for Saint Mikulas, and if they have been good, they receive sweets and toys. Naughty children receive only a bag of coal or potatoes from the Čert, while *very* bad children are told that he will put them into his sack and carry them off![21]

In Scandinavia, the house Elves known as Nisser must be fed on Christmas Eve or mayhem and mischief can result. The usual offering is a bowl of Rice porridge with a pat of butter, which should be left in a prominent spot, such as the barn.

In Cyprus, *xerotighna* pastry balls are tossed onto the roof at Christmas time to distract and appease evil Spirits. Like the Kallikantzaroi, the Spirits afflicting Cyprus are not that smart, and they will get confused trying to count the balls.[22]

Christmas Witches

And then there are the Christmas Witches, spiritual beings that may be seen as saints in one place and as Demons in another. Some regard the Witch figure as a benevolent force for healing (as in, for example, La Befana), while others find her (or him) terrifying. As one example, Lucia, the light bearer, whose holy day on December 13 is celebrated as the start of the Christmas season in Scandinavia, is regarded as a saint in Sicily and Sweden, but in Slovenia and Croatia she is known as "Dark Lutz" who scourges lazy girls and disembowels children who are truly bad. In Norway, Lucia is said to punish anyone who works on her special day.

The old woman Witch known in German and Austrian lore as Frau Berchta derives from the Norse Berchta, wife of Odin. She is reported to abduct children in one part of Germany but in other parts is a benevolent gift bringer who enters the rooms of children to comfort them and bring treats. She is sometimes said to lead the Wild Hunt, a gang of lost souls who fly across the winter sky on Christmas Eve, or she may bring gifts to those who assist her. If you are among those who fear her, it's best to protect yourself by eating fish and rolls on twelfth night—if you don't, she will cut open your body, fill it with chaff, and sew you up again with an iron chain!

Other precautions may need to be taken at this vulnerable time when dark powers roam the wintry landscape. Norwegians hide their brooms so that Witches aren't tempted to steal them and take them for a ride, and to prevent Witches from coming down the chimney, Yule Logs are left burning all night, salt is sprinkled on fires, and woods that tend to spark, like Spruce or Pine, are chosen for the hearth fire.

Austrians burn incense for protection and use brooms to "sweep away" any lurking evil forces during the Yule season, while in England the silverware is polished to a gleam so that evil Spirits and Witches will see their own face and be frightened away.[23]

As you can see, Witches exist very much in the eye of the beholder, and while there are some who fear them, there are others who will do everything in their power to make them feel welcome!

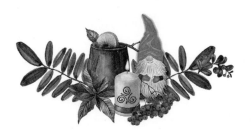

THE ANIMALS AT YULE

Christmas Eve, and twelve of the clock.
"Now they are all on their knees,"
An elder said as we sat in a flock
By the embers in hearthside ease.

THOMAS HARDY, "THE OXEN" (1915)

There is a folk legend that farm animals and pets can speak at midnight on Christmas Eve, based on the belief that Jesus was born in a barn at the stroke of midnight on that day, leading to a miracle of the animals. The deer of the forest are said to look up at the sky at exactly the same time, and the bees to hum, but, it's said, only the pure of heart can hear it.[1]

Whether in the barn, field, or forest, animals figure predominantly in many Yuletide traditions. In England, farmers once gave their cows and oxen extra-nice fodder and wassailed them (sang to them and anointed them with cider) to ensure the health of the herd. In Poland, farmers traditionally gave an *oplatek* (a simple flour-and-water wafer that resembles the wafers distributed at Christmas Mass) to their cows on Christmas Eve, and extra food to their horses on December 26. In northern Europe, the ancient Teutons sacrificed a white horse to their Gods at Yule.

In fact, horses are intimately associated with Yuletide. In Indo-European spirituality, the horse is a creature of the Sun and of Agni, sacred fire, so it is easy to see how ancient cultures would have built rituals around horses to hasten the return of the Sun in the darkest season. We'll look at some here.

The Mari Lwyd (Gray Mare)

In Wales, a man would dress as the Mari Lwyd (Gray Mare) and wander from house to house, escorted by a gang of guisers, between Christmas Day and Twelfth Night (January 5 or 6). The Mari Lwyd was a mare's skull affixed to a stick and decorated with ribbons and bells. The lower jaw of the skull clacked as if the mare were speaking, and the man holding it was covered with a blanket to disguise his human form.

Arriving at the door, the men would knock and ask to enter. A householder would welcome in the Mari, asking that she please not wreck the house. But once inside, the Mari would lunge at the welcoming housewife with her clacking jaws. The only way to stop the mayhem was for a small child to offer candy, and then the mare would suddenly go quiet.

As noted, in Indo-European culture, horses were considered solar animals, and welcoming the horse into the house was a way of letting in the strengthening light. The Mari would pay particular attention to the women of the house—especially unwed women, bringing the fertility of the Sun to them.

The color gray is liminal, symbolic of Solstice, which falls between the deepening dark of Samhain (Halloween) and the rekindled sunlight of Imbolc (Brighid's Day). The mare is the great Celtic symbol of sovereignty, of the Land Goddess who marries the ruler and without whom his reign has no legitimacy. Through ritual, the Mari Lwyd strengthens the community's ties to the Goddess of the Land by visiting every home.[2]

The Hooden Horse

"Hoodening" is another ancient winter tradition in Kent, England. A group of villagers go from pub to pub and house to house during the four days before Christmas, performing humorous plays, drinking beer, and collecting donations. The "Hooden Horse"—a creature that is exhausted from hard work forced on it by "the boss"—is a standard character in their performances.

Sometimes the Hooden Horse is accompanied by two other horses, and that's interesting because in Indo-European lore, three is a sacred number implying a high God or Goddess or an important divinity. The word *hooden* may derive from *wooden, hooded, hide* (as in an animal skin), or *hoaden* (a type of cloth), or it may even be a derivation of the name of Woden, the old Norse deity.[3]

A similar custom was once enacted in Cheshire, England, in which a man hidden under a sackcloth carried the head of a dead horse, called Old Hob, apparently in order to frighten people.[4]

The Laair Vane (White Horse)

The tradition of the Laair Vane comes from the Isle of Man. We have a description of the ritual from Manx historian A. W. Moore:

> During the supper the laare vane, or white mare, was brought in. This was a horse's head made of wood, and so contrived that the person who had charge of it, being concealed under a white sheet, was able to snap the mouth. He went round the table snapping the horse's mouth at the guests who finally chased him from the room, after much rough play. A similar custom is mentioned by Dr. Johnson as taking place on New Year's Eve, in Scotland: One of the company dressed himself in a cow's hide, upon which the rest of the party belaboured him with sticks. They all then left the house and ran round it, only being re-admitted on repeating the following words, which are still preserved in St. Kilda: "May God bless this house and all that belongs to it, cattle, stones and timber. In plenty of meat, of bed and body clothes, and health of men, may it ever abound." Each then pulled off a piece of the hide, and burnt it for the purpose of driving away disease. The Manx custom was probably formerly the same as this.[5]

The Christmas Bull

Very similar to the Welsh Mari Lwyd (the previous page), the tradition from the west of England, called the Christmas Bull or the Broad, features a man covered with a hide or sheet and carrying a bull's head mounted on a pole. If not an actual preserved bull's head, the head might be made of cardboard, with horns, glass eyes, ribbons, and rosettes attached.

The Christmas Bull may be part of a guising group (page 38), a wassailing team (page 114), or a hero-combat play. He is generally accompanied by ordinarily dressed handlers, who sometimes carry a wooden bowl of wassail, decorated with evergreens and ribbons. The group wanders from door to door as the Bull prances about, threatening the homeowners until given food and drink.[6]

Santa's Reindeer

Reindeer are another ubiquitous animal of the Yuletide season. They are said to pull Santa's sleigh and are found in ornaments and seasonal decorations of all kinds. But there is a pervasive misconception about the reindeer that pull Santa around the world. Despite popular lore, they are all female! Santa's reindeer can't be male for one simple reason: Only female reindeer still have antlers at the time of Christmas. The males of the species drop their antlers before mid-December. Female reindeer in winter are also larger than the males, having more body fat, which puts them at an advantage in terms of the endurance it takes to fly around the world.[7]

There is a theory about the origins of Santa Claus and his reindeer. Siberian reindeer like to feast on *Amanita muscaria* (Fly Agaric or Amanita), a mushroom that is red with white spots, grows in northern latitudes, and is a common feature of northern European Christmas decorations. Amanita is hallucinogenic and can be quite deadly to humans, so Siberian shamans (medicine men and women) would drink the urine of a reindeer that had eaten the mushrooms, allowing the shaman to use the mushroom to safely go into a healing trance. Is Santa Claus the plant Spirit of Amanita, just as Mescalito is to the Peyote cactus? Or is he just a depiction of a Siberian shaman tripping with the reindeer?

Substantiating evidence for that theory comes from the fact that Siberian shamans would visit people's homes and give them bags of dried red Amanita as gifts. Amanita is also strongly associated with

Pine trees because the mushrooms like to grow under them. Could this be the origin of the Christmas tree? And Rudolph (who, as we have seen, must have been a female) has a bright red nose. Is this another Amanita reference? And, of course, Santa lives at the North Pole, where the reindeer and the shamans dwell.[8]

Of course, it's not always reindeer that pull Santa's sleigh. In Australia, six male kangaroos are said to pull Father Christmas around, while in the Netherlands, he rides upon a white horse, and in Switzerland, he gets around on a donkey. As noted earlier, in some traditions in Louisiana, he is drawn by alligators—and a werewolf with a red nose![9]

The Hunting of the Wren

In its earliest version, the Celtic Hunting of the Wren ceremony was always held on "Wren Day," December 26. It started with the pursuit of a live wren that was killed with stones. Then the dead bird was placed in a decorated box or cage ornamented with ribbons, evergreens, and fruits and was paraded through the town by a procession of "Wren Boys," accompanied by musicians, dancers, singers, and guisers. The guisers would traditionally include the characters of Cailleach (the Old Hag and queen of winter) and a Láir Bhán (White Mare) as the group moved from house to house, looking for money to "bury the wren."

In the end, the dead wren, an omen of bad luck, was deposited on the land of the most miserly and ungenerous household the group had encountered. But sometimes, instead, it would be buried in a liminal place, such as a shoreline. Such places were betwixt and between, "thin places" between land and water, between this world and the Otherworld. (The magical area of a shoreline is between the row of tide-tossed seaweed and the water. Known as the "black shore," it is a powerful place to do ceremonies.)

The collected funds, of course, went toward celebratory food and drink, and sometimes the wren boys carried a bowl or wassail, from which onlookers could sip for a small donation.[10]

The Wran! The Wran! The King of all birds,
St. Stephen's Day was caught in the furze.
Although he is little his honor is great,
So rise up young lady and give us a trate.

We followed this wran three miles or more,
Through hedges and ditches and frost and snow,
We knocked him down and we broke his knee,
And we brought him home on a holly tree.

Holly and Ivy well sot up,
The man of the house was in very good luck,
A bottle of whisky and a glass of beer,
And we wish you all a happy New Year.

So now young lady shake up your feathers,
And do not think that we are beggars.
We are the boys who came today
To bury the wran on St. Stephen's Day.

Up with the kirtle and down with the pan,
Give us our answer and let us be gone.

TRADITIONAL IRISH RHYME FOR ST. STEPHEN'S DAY

But why did they pick on the poor little wren? According to Druidic teachings, the wren is known as the "Druid bird." The story is this: One day the birds had a contest to see which of them could fly the highest and claim the title of "king of the birds." The mighty goose, the wily raven, the wise owl, the swift falcon, and many other birds joined in the competition. The eagle, full of confidence in its powerful wings, easily flew higher than the others, sailing majestically through the clouds. The eagle flew and flew until, exhausted, it could fly no higher. At that exact moment a tiny wren popped out of the eagle's feathers, where it had been hiding all along. The wren shot straight up into the sky, proving that it could fly higher than any bird, including the mighty eagle.

In this way, the tiny wren showed that brains, more than muscle, make one a truly powerful ruler. And, like the wren, the Druids relied on memory and intelligence more than physical strength. So, the Druids claimed the wren as the "Druid bird," even using their calls as divinations (see below). It was also sometimes known as the "Witches' bird" because its feathers were protective against sorcery.

In later Christian times, then, the wren may have been hunted because it was seen as a symbol of the Druidic art, or perhaps simply to show contempt for magic and divination.

In the modern era, there are still dances and parades to honor the wren, and celebrants carry a staff decorated with ribbons. Thankfully, no wrens are killed, and proceeds of the day are donated to charity.

Here are the prognostications that were once taken from the calls of the wren:

- If it called from the east, pious visitors were approaching with discourtesy toward you.
- If from the southeast, proud jesters were approaching.
- If from the southwest, ex-freemen were coming.
- If from the northeast, women were coming.
- If from the northwest, pious folk were on their way.
- If from the south, and provided the calls were not between you and the Sun, someone dear to you would be slain or unfaithful.
- If at your left ear, it meant sexual union with a young person.
- If from behind you, another person was pursuing your spouse.
- If from on the ground behind you, your spouse would be taken by force.
- If from the east, poets were coming or bringing a message.
- If from behind you from the south, the heads of good clergy were coming, or tidings of the death of noble clergy.
- If from the southwest, robbers, evil peasants, or bad women were coming toward you.
- If from the west, wicked relations were coming.
- If from the northwest, a noble hero, a good woman, or a generous person was coming.

- If from the north, bad people or wicked youths were approaching.
- If from the south, it meant sickness and wolves.
- If from the ground, a stone, or a cross, it meant the death tidings of a great man.
- If from many crosses, it meant a great slaughter of men, and the number of times the wren alighted on the ground would give the numbers of the dead.[11]

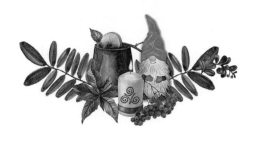

Rituals and Rites of Solstice, Yule, and Christmas

Christmas and Yule have long been times for make-believe, guising, mumming, and wearing disguises. It is an interval of permissiveness when revelers don straw masks and gender-bending clothing. This shape-shifting attire, merrymaking, and traveling among houses are reminders that the Spirits are active at the Solstice, bringing both chaos and the gifts of the season. The yearly repetition of time-honored customs is assurance that the community will be protected as the world waits for spring.

First Footing

In Scotland, Wales, and other parts of Europe, the "First Footing" is a type of magical practice designed to bring luck in the New Year and at Christmas. In essence, the first person to cross the threshold of the house after the stroke of midnight on Christmas Eve or on New Year's Eve determines the fortunes of the family in the year to come.

Typically, the most desirable visitor is a dark, handsome, single male, especially if he has a high arched foot or was born feet first. Undesirable visitors are those with flat feet, those whose eyebrows grow together over their nose, and blond or red-haired men or women (which makes me think this might be a tribal memory of Viking marauders!).

In some areas, having a woman as the first visitor spells serious trouble for the house and could bring birth defects or even death to the family. At Hogmanay (New Year's Eve), Scottish families have been known to push a dark-haired young man outside and force him to wait until midnight to come back in, just so he will be the first one to cross the doorway!

The First Footer is supposed to bring a present, make a toast to the house, or feed the fire (in Scotland, he often arrives with a bottle of whiskey in hand). He or she should go in by the front door and leave by the back door, because opening the doors "lets the new year in."

In eastern Europe, the First Footer brings a bouquet of Wheat at dawn on Christmas Eve day and sprinkles the grain over the family, blesses the house, pounds the fire hard enough to make sparks, and then stays for the feast. He leaves that night with a gift.

For the Greeks, it is very important that the First Footer come in with their right foot first. The custom is known as *podariko* (good foot) and closely resembles the Scottish custom of First Footing. Entering with the right foot first brings health and good luck to the home. The First Footer is given treats after they come through the door, and then the homeowner steps on a piece of iron to ground the luck and to ensure strength and health to the family.[1]

In Wales, the very worst omen is having a red-haired woman be first through the door after midnight on New Year's Eve. A dark-haired man, on the other hand, is a good omen. If the First Footer happens to be female, boys are required to run around in the house to undo the damage. This practice, known as "breaking the Witch," is supposed to break any spell or malign influence brought in by a woman who just might be a Witch.[2]

Guising and Mumming at Yuletide

To mask and to mum kind neighbours will come
With wassails of nut-brown ale,
To drink and carouse to all in the house,
As merry as bucks in the dale;

Where cake, bread and cheese is brought for your fees,
To make you the longer stay;
At the fire to warm will do you no harm,
To drive the cold winter away.

"ALL HAIL TO THE DAYS,"
AN ENGLISH CAROL (CA. 1625)

Perhaps echoing the appearance of Spirits that roam the land in winter, in many communities there was once a tradition of guisers and mummers going house to house in costume, merrymaking and begging for coins or treats. The practice may have been a way of enforcing generosity in the coldest season, of reinforcing neighborly ties, and of reassuring everyone that they could depend on food and good cheer to tide them over to the warmer days ahead.

The historical origins of persons going about in costumes and gender-bending attire is recorded as far back as the Roman Saturnalia revels. As Gerry Bowler tells us in the *World Encyclopedia of Christmas:*

> In 1445 the Paris Faculty of Theology complained, "Priests and clerks may be seen wearing masks and monstrous visages at the hours of office. They dance in the choir dressed as women, panders, or minstrels." The Staffordshire [England] Horn Dance has a cross-dressing cast member called Maid Marian, while guising on the Scottish borders provides comic relief with the figure of Bessie the Besom, a man dressed as an old woman.[3]

During the twelve days of Christmas on the Shetland Islands, one might see *skeklers* or *guliks:* guisers who dressed in straw costumes and conical hats, with handkerchiefs covering their faces. They would fire a shot when approaching a farm, and if there was an answering shot, they would visit the home. There they would dance and be given refreshments and coins.

In eastern Scotland, guisers wore straw hats and ribbons and blackened their faces. If a door was left open, they considered themselves invited in, and they would try to steal a kiss from any female in the lodging.[4]

Some parts of Nova Scotia once had a similar custom called

Belsnickeling, based on the name of the German masked, fur-clad fig-ure named Belsnickel who accompanies Saint Nicholas on his rounds (see page 20). A group of people dressed in costume and carrying bells and chains visited their neighbors, who would try to guess the identity of each Belsnickel.[5]

Belsnickeling had migrated to the United States with early German settlers, including the Pennsylvania Deutsch. Here women sometimes played the role. Masked figures dressed in rags would appear at a home, banging on the door and windows, demanding entry. Once inside, they threw sweets on the floor. As the children bent to grab the sweets, the Belsnickelers would smack them with a switch as punishment for their greed. In other cases, the guisers performed some entertainment and were given "payment" of hot chocolate, sweets, whiskey, or moonshine. If the homeowner correctly guessed their identity, they removed their mask.

Here is one account of the American tradition from the nineteenth century in Allegany County, Maryland, where women sometimes played the part:

> He was known as Kriskinkle, Beltznickle and sometimes as the Christmas woman. Children then not only saw the mysterious person, but felt him or rather his stripes upon their backs with his switch. The annual visitor would make his appearance some hours after dark, thoroughly disguised, especially the face, which would sometimes be covered with a hideously ugly phiz—generally wore a female garb—hence the name Christmas woman—sometimes it would be a veritable woman but with masculine force and action. He or she would be equipped with an ample sack about the shoul-ders filled with cakes, nuts, and fruits, and a long hazel switch which was supposed to have some kind of a charm in it as well as a sting. One hand would scatter the goodies upon the floor, and then the scramble would begin by the delighted children, and the other hand would ply the switch upon the backs of the excited youngsters—who would not show a wince, but had it been parental discipline there would have been screams to reach a long distance.[6]

Shanghaiing was a Scotch-Irish and German tradition in which mummers dressed in costumes and rode around on decorated buggies, horses, and mules. They would halt in front of a house to sing and make noise, but they didn't enter, because the whole idea was just to have fun. The conservative religious groups common in these communities, such as the Mennonites and Brethren, frowned upon the tradition because of its supposed Pagan roots. Most Belsnickeling customs died out after World War II.[7]

In Wales, in a tradition called Calenning ("a little gift" or "the first day of the month," deriving from the Latin *kalends*), boys went door to door bearing a clove-studded orange or apple. In his 1924 collection of essays, *Dog and Duck,* Welsh author Arthur Machen recalls:

When I was a boy . . . there was a very queer celebration on New Year's Day in the little Monmouthshire town where I was born, Caerleon-on-Usk. The town children . . . got the biggest and bravest and gayest apple they could find in the loft, deep in the dry bracken. They put bits of gold leaf upon it. They stuck raisins into it. They inserted into the apple little sprigs of box, and then they delicately slit the ends of hazel nuts, and so worked that the nuts appeared to grow from the ends of the box-leaves. . . . At last, three bits of stick were fixed into the base of the apple, tripod-wise; and so it was borne round from house to house; and the children got cakes and sweets, and—those were wild days, remember—small cups of ale.[8]

The Calenning fruit was kept in the house as a good luck charm all year, and the custom persisted until the 1980s.[9]

Silvesterchläusen is the tradition of Old Silvester (commemorating the death of Pope Sylvester I) on New Year's Eve (December 31) and Old New Year's Eve (January 13) in Switzerland. Starting at dawn, groups of men visit households wearing costumes and ringing bells. Some dress as *die Wüeschten* (the ugly), covered in pine branches, cedar branches, or straw, large cowbells, and ugly masks with googly eyes, ferocious teeth, and sometimes horns. *Die Schönen* (the beautiful) wear brightly colored traditional women's alpine dress and giant headdresses depicting entire miniature landscapes. *Die Schön-Wüeschten* (the beautiful-ugly) wear costumes made of forest elements, like the ugly, but with masks that are more human in appearance. Their headpieces are made of twigs, leaves, nuts, and straw, with an iconic mask of pine cones. Their elaborate headwear depicts alpine scenes such as barns.

Neighbors open their doors when the *Chläuse* (the Silvesterchläusen mummers) appear, offering food, snacks, and warm drinks to anyone who enters the home. The origins of the tradition are murky. Some think the rustic costumes and bell ringing are meant to scare away evil Spirits to make the way clear for a happy and prosperous new year. Clergy, of course, long decried it as a Pagan custom.[10]

In the German Buttenmandelhaut (Riddle-Raddle Man) tradition, masked men covered in straw disguises burst into the barn, ringing cowbells and shaking rattles. A Saint Nicholas figure blesses them, the farmer's wife sprinkles them with holy water, and they set out, proceeding from door to door with presents for children. If they happen to encounter an unmarried woman, they will pick her up and carry her outside. The whole pageant appears to be yet another instance of using loud noises to scare away evil Spirits of the old year and of winter. The "blessing" by Saint Nicholas seems to be a way of making the ritual acceptable to the church.[11]

The Yule Log

Come, bring with a noise,
My merry, merry boys,
The Christmas Log to the firing;
While my good Dame, she
Bids ye all be free;
And drink to your heart's desiring.
With the last year's brand
Light the new block, and
For good success in his spending,
On your Psalteries play,
That sweet luck may

Come while the log is a-tinding.
Drink now the strong beer,
Cut the white loaf here,
The while the meat is a-shredding;
For the rare mince-pie
And the plums stand by
To fill the paste that's a-kneading.

ROBERT HERRICK, "CEREMONIES FOR
CHRISTMAS," SEVENTEENTH CENTURY

For millions of years we humans have regarded fire as a source of comfort and protection. We cooked our food, told our stories, and danced around fire. Fire heated our homes, and bonfires kept predators away from the herds in calving and lambing seasons. When we wished to offer up a prayer seeking comfort, help, or support, we would light a candle, a small, personal fire. Fire carried our wishes and needs to the heavens, where the powers we worshipped might yet hear our pleas.

The Yule Log is a special kind of fire, a long-lasting, continuous ritual blaze that protects the home during the most frightening time of year. The tradition of burning a large piece of wood in the hearth during the Winter Solstice and Christmas season was first known in the Italian Alps, Balkans, Scandinavia, France, and Iberia. Britain adopted the custom later (except for Lowland Scotland, where it was suppressed by Calvinist Protestants). In essence, the Yule Log burns continuously in the hearth—which, other than key holes, is the only vulnerable opening of the home where mischievous Spirits might enter—through the twelve days of Christmas (Christmas Day through the evening of January 5— known as twelfth night). By saving a piece of the log all year, the family carries the protection through to the next Yuletide. A piece of the Yule Log is saved to kindle the next year's Yule Log, also a way of carrying over good luck and protection from one year to the next.

In England, Oak is the traditional wood for a Yule Log, while in France it is Cherry and in Scotland it is Birch. In ancient times, the Yule Log might sometimes be an entire tree—the trunk was dragged into the house and the butt end pushed into the fireplace. As it gradually burned through the twelve days of Christmas, from Christmas Day through the evening of January 5, or Twelfth Night, it was repeatedly driven deeper into the hearth.[12]

The customs embedded in the Yule Log ritual differed from place to place. In France, families went out together to seek the Buche de Noel (Christmas log), while in Norway, the father of the house performed this duty. In England, the log was selected at Candlemas (February 1–2) and set aside to dry for the next Yule celebration, while in Serbia it was cut in the dark early on Christmas Eve morning and transported by candlelight to the house that evening. In the United States, it was considered good luck to harvest the log from one's own property.

The log might be carried or dragged into the house in high spirits and decorated with ribbons, leaves, and even flowers, if such could be found. Bread might be laid upon the log or juniper placed under it. Coins might be placed on top and then given away for luck. The smallest revelers might hitch a ride as it was pulled across the snow. Once the log crossed the threshold, it might be sprinkled with grain and spirits. In some traditions, the head of the family took a drink of wine, passed the cup to all family members, and then poured the remaining liquid onto the log three times. The family might carry the log three times around the kitchen (which is, after all, the central hearth-fire of the home) before laying it in the fireplace and kindling it with a piece of last year's log.

It is worth noting that these traditions carry symbolic weight. Bread and grain carry the luck of the harvest and the protective energy of the Sun. Coins are also solar symbols. Juniper is an herb of immortality (because it is an evergreen) and of purification. Alcoholic spirits are liquids of fire, bringing the promise and blessings of the hot Sun to the darkest and coldest days.

In Germany the log was placed in the hearth on Christmas Eve or Christmas Day and only lightly burned. It was kept all year, and when storms threatened, this now magical log was set alight as protection.

In the Scottish Highlands, a twisted stump or root was carried home on Christmas Eve and carved into the figure of an old woman, the Cailleach Nollaig (Christmas Hag or Goddess). The Cailleach was burned in the hearth to protect the home from misfortune.[13]

In Scandinavia, huge bonfires were once lit to entice the Sun to return and to honor the God Thor as part of the Jól (Yule) festival, and the Yule fire was said to purify the home of evil forces.

In Latvia, some ancient Pagan midwinter customs are still maintained, such as "the rolling of the log," for which an Oak is cut down and sawn into sections, and one piece is dragged around the house and land before being burned in the hearth. The Oak log symbolizes eternal life, and burning it is said to call back and strengthen light and the Sun. The log also burns off any bad luck lingering in the neighborhood.[14]

In various traditions, once the Yule Log was burned, its ashes might be mixed with the cow's fodder, as the cinders were believed to aid the cows in giving birth. When mixed with soil, the ashes helped the crops, and when dropped in a well, they were said to purify the water. In Serbia and Croatia, a log of Oak (the *badnjak*) is burned on Christmas Eve, and a piece of it is saved and placed in the branch of a fruit tree to ensure fertility.

Other Yuletide Rituals of Fire

Yule Logs, bonfires, candles lit in windows, and the strings of twinkling electrical lights we hang on our homes and trees today are a faint memory of the winter fire festivals and rituals our ancestors once cherished—and relied on for protection against the cold, the dark, and the roaming Spirits of winter. Here, we'll look at some whose stories have survived through history.

The Yule Candle
Sometimes, in place of a Yule Log, householders might burn a candle. In England, a Yule candle would be kept lit for all of Christmas Day to bring good luck. In Scandinavia, the candle was burned all night on Christmas Eve. The stub of the candle was then rubbed on the plow and on animals and kept as a talisman to protect the house from storms.

The Ashen Fagot

> *The pondrous ashen faggot, from the yard,*
> *The jolly farmer to his crowded hall*
> *Conveys, with speed; where, on the rising flames*
> *(Already fed with store of massy brands)*
> *It blazes soon; nine bandages it bears,*
> *And as they each disjoin (so custom wills),*
> *A mighty jug of sparkling cyder's brought,*
> *With brandy mixt, to elevate the guests.*
>
> ROMAINE JOSEPH THORN, "CHRISTMAS" (1795)

The Ashen fagot is an English Yule Log custom that most likely has Viking roots. *Ashen* refers to the Ash tree, which is regarded as Yggdrasil, the Tree of Life or World Tree in Norse mythology, while a *fagot* is a bundle—in this case, a bundle of ash sticks.

For the ritual, a bundle of Ash sticks was bound with lengths of green Ash bands, sometimes called beams, preferably all from the same tree. The bundle could be huge—as long as twelve feet, bound with twelve or more bands. It would be set in the hearth and lit with a piece saved from the previous year's bundle, preferably by the oldest person in the room.

As the bundle burned, the bands would break in the fire. A toast was drunk each time a band broke. Unmarried women might each pick a band, and the one whose band burned first would be the first to marry.

Folklore held that any household that did not burn the Ashen fagot would face years of bad luck and misfortune. Some versions suggest that an Ashen fagot kept in the house would ward away evil Spirits.[15]

Up Helly Aa

In the Shetland Islands, on the last Tuesday in January, even up to the present day, the Up Helly Aa (Up Holy Day) festival features men in Viking costumes accompanied by marching bands carrying a model of a Viking longship through town. At the end of the procession, the Viking ship is set on fire as ships at anchor in the harbor sound their sirens and the crowd cheers. This act marks the official end of the Yule season.

The Burning of the Clavie

The Burning of the Clavie on January 11 (the old date of New Year's, before the introduction of the Julian calendar) at Burghead, on the Moray Firth in Scotland, is another fire festival with ancient origins. The Church of Scotland declared it "superstitious, idolatrous and sinful" and "an abominable heathenish practice" in 1714, but nevertheless, it became a firmly entrenched celebration of Hogmanay (Scottish New Year's).

The *clavie* (a wooden barrel filled with tar and staves) is mounted on a pole, set afire, and carried around town, accompanied by a large crowd, finally ending up atop Doorie Hill on the ramparts of an old Pictish fort. Here it is sent rolling down the hill, and as it goes, onlookers eagerly gather up the still smoldering embers. Possession of a piece of the *clavie* is said to bring good luck in the new year.[16]

Rauhnächte

The twelve nights of Christmas, starting December 21, are a liminal time between the lunar year, which comprises 354 days, and the solar year, which comprises 365 days. In Austria, this magical interlude is traditionally seen as a time when the laws of nature can be overturned. It is said that one's fate can be changed during this time, and the dead are said to roam the Earth, whispering prophecies to those who are sensitive enough to hear.

In the ritual known as the Rauhnächte (Smoke Nights), guisers dressed as Witches and Demons roam the streets, sweeping the steps and stables with their brooms as families burn herbal incense in their homes to ward off evil Spirits. Dried herbs with protective properties, such as Mugwort, Ferns, Sage, and Cedar are mixed with Frankincense and burned on charcoal briquettes. The fumigation starts at the oven, then moves to each corner of the kitchen, then to the outer rooms of the house, and finally farther out into the stables and farm. The carrying of smoke outward from the stove is a way of spreading the warmth of the sacred hearth throughout the house and land, laying a magical blanket of protection against the cold and evil Spirits.

Blessings are spoken as the smoke purifies the home and land. For example:

May everything that is dark, everything that no longer
   serves us,
disappear from this room.
We invite in love, light, and blessings.
May this room shine with a new, fresh, and brilliant luster,
peace, serenity, and strength.
Thank you.*

A final precaution against evil Spirits that might be lurking is that bedding and laundry are not supposed to be hung or aired outside at this time, because noxious forces could get tangled up in the linens.[17]

Divinations at Yuletide

Such winters as are void of snow, are not so good for the fruits of the ground, as more snowie winters. Whereupon Plinie affirmeth, that he which saith clear winters are to be wished, wisheth no good for the trees and plants: and in that regard your experienced husbandman desireth that the winter may be cold and snowie, rather then clear and warm: For besides this they also say, that a hot Christmas makes a fat Church-yard.

JOHN SWAN, *SPECULUM MUNDI: OR A GLASSE*
REPRESENTING THE FACE OF THE WORLD (1643)

As the new year approaches it is a time of celebration and also a time of anxiety as to what kind of blessings or disappointments the coming year will bring. The time of dissolution and chaos between the old year and the new is a liminal time when spiritual energies and forces are more easily tapped. Omens and portents are sought and predictions made.

Weather Divination
Making predictions based on the weather is common at Christmas and New Year's. For example, a green Christmas (or a warm winter)

---

*When doing smudging or smoke purification, please remember to crack a window or a door somewhere in the house so the "nasties" can escape.

means that the graveyards will fill up. This is true because a cold winter means that bacteria and other pests that cause disease will die, and also that plants can grow properly in the next season. There is nothing worse for a tree or bush than to put out new shoots or flowers in a warm winter, only to have them wither in a sudden spate of freezing weather.

Other forms of divination dealt with predicting the weather based on signs and symbols. If the Holly produced a large crop of berries, for example, it was said that the winter would be hard. England once had a tradition of weather and harvest forecasting based on the day of the week that Christmas fell on. Here are some of those prognostications:

Sunday: It means a warm winter and a hot, dry, and fair summer. Sheep and honey will do well. Fruits and gardens will flourish, but old men will die, as will women with child. Married folks will be at peace.

Monday: It means a misty winter and a windy and stormy summer. The harvest will be good, but there will be little honey. Bees will die, and women will mourn for their husbands.

Tuesday: It means the winter will be cold and moist, with much snow. Summer will be wet, with a poor harvest. Swine and other animals will die. Kings and princes will get along well, but clergy will perish.

Wednesday: It means winter will be sharp and hard, but the harvest will be good, with plenty of hay, wine, and corn. There will be a lack of honey and fruit, and cattle, young people, and children will die.

Thursday: It means winter will be windy and good, and summer will be rainy and cold. There will be a good harvest, but not much honey. Great men will die, while governors and kings will be at peace.

Friday: It means winter will be steadfast, but the harvest will be poor. There will be plenty of wine and corn, and hay will be good, but sheep and bees will die. People will suffer eye pains, and there will be fruit, but children will get sick.

Saturday: It means winter will be misty, with much snow. Summer will be dry, with a poor harvest. There will be little corn and fruit, but pastures will be good. There will be war in many countries, with sickness. The old will die, trees will wither, and bees will pass away.[18]

Marriage Divination

According to British tradition, "the flower of the well" is the first water drawn from a well in the new year, and it was said to bring special luck. If a woman was the first to draw water, she would be married within the year. Giving the first water to the cows guaranteed more milk, and kept in a bottle, the water protected the house.

Divination and Rituals to Bring Back the Sun

In Russia, there is a type of Christmas divination known as Podblyudnuiya in which small tokens—such as copper, silver, or golden rings—are dropped into a bowl that is then covered with a cloth. Songs are sung, and at the end of each song one person reaches into the bowl and pulls out a token, and a divination is made. When the songs are finished, a game called "the burial of the gold" begins: The last gold ring left in the bowl is taken up by a young woman, who walks around the circle with it in her fingers. She slips the ring into someone's hand, and then the ring is passed around from person to person as quickly as possible. There is singing all the while, and when the song ends the young woman has to guess whose hands the ring is in.

The game of finding the golden ring may be symbolic of recovering the lost sunlight. Bonfires in the Russian landscape are also common at this time, which may be a magical way to strengthen the returning solar light and warmth.[19]

In Ukraine, Saint Andrew's Day, which falls on December 13 of the Orthodox calendar, is traditionally celebrated with fortune-telling and mischievous pranks, such as putting a plow on a house roof, hiding someone's fence, or taking a gate off its hinges.[20] In the evening, young men and women play a game with *kalyta* bread, a dry, flat, round loaf with a hole in its center that is decorated with Poppy seeds, dried Cherries, or Raisins. The women hide the bread, and the men have to guess where it is. After much joking and horseplay, the girls eventually reveal the location of the bread, which is then smeared with golden honey and hung in the middle of the house. Everyone tries their best to grab a mouthful as the host of the night swings the *kalyta,* making it hard for anyone to snatch a bite. Afterward, everyone sits at the dinner table and shares a meal.

The rituals connected with the round, honey-smeared kalyta bread may have been connected to the birth of the new Sun after the Winter Solstice. After the conversion to Christianity, the bread rituals were moved to the feast day of Saint Andrew.[21]

Divinations for Luck and Friendship

In Spain and Italy, in a ritual called the "urn of fate," enacted at Christmas time, pairs of names are pulled out of a jar. Those named are destined to be friends all year long.

In Brazil, African folk tradition and Catholicism merge in the festival of the Goddess Lemanjá. On New Year's Eve, devotees head to the beach and scatter gifts for her on the water. If the offerings drift out to sea, it means she has taken them and good luck will follow. If they drift back to shore, a sad year lies ahead.[22]

Divinatory Cakes and Puddings

"Christmas pudding" or "Plum pudding" is a round, boiled English dessert that is served flaming with brandy and garnished with a sprig of Holly for Christmas. The concept is derived from the medieval boiled dinners served to nobility, which were made from meat and fruits, especially Plums, and were known as a "Plum pottage."

A ring, a button, a thimble, or a coin might be hidden inside the Plum pudding. Each token tells the fate of the person who finds it: marriage (the ring), spinsterhood or bachelorhood (the thimble), or wealth in the coming year (the coin). Ideally, the pudding is made from thirteen ingredients; for Christians, that number represents the twelve apostles and Jesus, while for Pagans it represents the thirteen moons of the year. Each member of the family should take a turn stirring the ingredients, from east to west, and it's said that anyone who does not take at least one bite will lose a friend in the new year. (See page 66 for a traditional Christmas pudding recipe.)

In Scandinavia, an Almond is hidden in a Rice pudding served at Christmas, and whoever finds the Almond must complete a task, such as inventing a rhyme of thanks for the meal.

In Ukraine, Poland, and Russia, the Christmas dish is the grain pudding called *kutia* (from the ancient Greek *kukkia*, "boiled grain"), which is made with Wheat berries, Poppy seeds, honey, nuts, and spices (see the recipe below). The grain symbolizes eternal life and rebirth, the poppy seeds are for fertility, and the honey for pleasure. The dish is shared with livestock and poultry as well as the humans of the family, for luck. The stickier the dish the better, because the head of the family takes a spoonful and tosses it up. The number of grains of porridge that stick to the ceiling tells how many sheaves of grain will be collected that year. An unmarried woman might take the first spoonful of *kutia*, wrap it in men's trousers, and then hide the bundle under a pillow in order to dream of her future husband.[23]

The Gateau des Roi (King's Cake) or Bean Cake was invented in the thirteenth century in Normandy, France, and served through the Middle Ages. A bean or a pea was hidden inside the cake, which was cut into as many pieces as there were guests. A child handed out the pieces, and whoever found the bean or pea in their piece was named king or queen of the celebration.[24] (See page 101 for a recipe.)

Now, now the mirth comes,
With the cake full of plums,
Where bean's the king of the sport here;
Beside we must know,
The pea also
Must revel, as queen, in the court here.

Begin then to choose,
This night as ye use,
Who shall for the present delight here,
Be a king by the lot,
And who shall not
Be Twelfth-day queen for the night here.

Which known, let us make
Joy-sops with the cake;
and let not a man then be seen here,
Who unurg'd will not drink
To the base from the brink
A health to the king and queen here.

ROBERT HERRICK, "TWELFTH NIGHT"
(SEVENTEENTH CENTURY)

🍲 Kutia: Christmas Wheat Berry Pudding

Makes 6–8 servings

1½ cups organic wheat berries

4½ cups organic milk, plus more as needed*

¾ cup poppy seeds

3 cups water

²/₃ cup slivered almonds or chopped walnuts

½ cup raw, local honey

²/₃ cup organic dried apricots, chopped

½ cup organic raisins

¹/₈ teaspoon sea salt

Rinse the wheat berries in cold water, then put them in a pan, add enough lukewarm water to cover them by at least 2 inches, and let them soak overnight. This step is important to soften the berries for cooking.

The next day, drain the wheat berries, put them in a medium pot, add the milk, and bring just to a boil over high heat. When the milk starts to boil, immediately reduce the heat to low, cover the pot, and simmer (do not boil) until the wheat berries are very tender and have split open, 3½ to 4 hours, depending on the quality of the wheat. Stir occasionally to prevent sticking.

Adapted from Natasha Kravchuk's "Kutia Recipe (Sweet Wheat Berry Pudding)," *Natasha's Kitchen* (blog), January 4, 2015.

---

*In some traditions, it's customary to avoid eating animal products on Christmas Eve. So, if you're making this on Christmas Eve, you can use water to make this *kutia,* if you prefer (though milk tastes better). The milk version is fine for Christmas Day.

Add more milk as needed to keep the wheat berries fully submerged.

While the wheat berries are simmering, rinse the poppy seeds in a fine-mesh sieve. Combine the rinsed poppy seeds with the water in a medium saucepan over medium heat. Bring the seeds just to a simmer (do not boil!), then remove from the heat, cover, and let sit for 30 minutes.

Return the poppy seed pan to a simmer (do not boil!), then, again, cover and let it sit for 30 minutes.

Drain the poppy seeds well through a sieve or cheesecloth. Then run them through a food grinder, using the fine grinding plate (or mill the poppy seeds in batches in a clean coffee grinder or, in a pinch, a mortar and pestle).

Preheat the oven to 350°F.

Spread the nuts on a baking sheet and toast in the oven for 5 minutes, then set aside and reduce the oven temperature to 325°F.

When the wheat berries are very tender and have split open, drain off the milk into a glass measuring cup. Keep ½ cup of the milk and discard the rest.

Combine the honey with the reserved milk and stir until well mixed.

Place the cooked wheat berries in a mixing bowl and add the ground poppy seeds, toasted nuts, honey-milk mixture, apricots, raisins, and salt. Stir everything together well, transfer to a casserole or pie dish, and bake for 20 minutes, uncovered.

Remove the *kutia* from the oven, cover it with aluminum foil, and let it rest for 15 minutes.

Serve warm or cold. The longer it sits, the more flavorful it will become. *Kutia* will keep in the fridge for about 2 weeks.

Taking the Greenery Down

Yuletide greenery, according to one tradition, should be taken down by Twelfth Night (January 5, the Eve of Epiphany) because any leftover leaf can become the abode of a goblin. As seventeenth-century poet Robert Herrick wrote:

> *Down with the rosemary, and so*
> *Down with the bay and mistletoe;*
> *Down with the holly, ivy, all*

Wherewith ye dress'd the Christmas Hall:
That so the superstitious find
No one least branch there left behind;
For look, how many leaves there be
Neglected, there (maids, trust to me),
So many goblins you shall see.[25]

On that same night, the Yule Log is removed from the hearth, and its ashes are mixed with the seeds for the spring planting. On Twelfth Day itself, an Epiphany cake is eaten, with a small token hidden inside. The finder becomes the king or queen of the day's festivities.

A different tradition holds that Imbolc (Candlemas), February 1 and 2, is the time when all Yuletide greenery should be swept from the house. The greenery is burned and a new Yule Log is selected, cut, and put aside to dry for the next year's festivities.[26]

❋ A Rite for the Goddess at the Winter Solstice

Here is a Winter Solstice rite that I composed for the Tribe of the Oak Druids (Tuatha na Dara) in honor of the Cailleach, known in some Celtic traditions as the Great Hag and winter face of the Land Goddess.

Before you perform a ritual to honor the Goddess at Winter Solstice, please make an offering to your local Land Spirits (it is only polite to make offerings to the Fairies, Elves, and Elementals that have helped you in your garden and home whenever you have a celebration). Here are some examples of things to offer them in winter:

- Make offerings to and sing to trees, especially fruit trees that have fed you all year.
- Hang fruits, bags of birdseed, and pine cones smeared with peanut butter and rolled in birdseed on the trees for the Spirits of the forest.
- Pour wine, honey, cider, or milk in the fields and on stones.
- Recite poetry for the trees.
- On Twelfth Night, hang toast in the branches of Apple trees, and pour cider made from the Apples of that orchard over their roots to give them a drink.
- Shout and make noise to wake up the Spirits and drive away blight.

- Put out a dish of cookies or oatmeal with a pat of butter, milk, and honey (or milk and whiskey), or a dish of mashed Potatoes with butter on top as an offering for the Fairies.

Note: Never put out chocolate, as it is toxic to many animals.

Create the Altar

Cover the altar with a faded tartan cloth or thick wool, and spread over it objects that speak of the winter season: rocks and crystals (maybe even sprinkled or washed with glitter to emulate frost), candles (white, black, blue, and gray), and anything else that evokes frost and snow. A small bough from an evergreen, such as Pine or Boxwood, would be a nice addition, as would any of the magical herbs of the Winter Solstice season.

Give a Welcome Statement

Your opening welcome might go something like this:

We are here to honor the Gods and to pay homage to the
Great Goddess of winter, An Cailleach, the Veiled One,
who haunts the frozen ground and the
frost-rimmed branches.
Her breath is the winter wind, her tears are the sleet,
and her skin is the snowbound field.
Great Hag of the gusty white rivers and fields,
we honor you and we welcome you!
All nature pauses under your gaze. Thank you for
this time of rest and purification!

Cleanse the Ritual Space

Begin by burning herbs of purification to cleanse your ritual space and all celebrants. Juniper was the herb of choice for purification in many European regions. If smoke is a problem, make an herbal brew and spray it on those attending the ritual and around the ceremonial area.

Light the Fire

Next bring the light of sacred fire into your ritual circle; light your bonfire if you're outdoors, or light a cauldron of candles or a fire in the hearth if you're indoors. Make offerings to the fire, such as butter, ghee, oil, whiskey, dried Mint, Cinnamon sticks, or other dried herbs, and anything else a fire would like. (If you're indoors, please remember to disengage your smoke alarms!)

Invoke Manannán MacLir to Open the Gates between the Worlds

Oh God of the headlands and Son of the Sea,
Manannán MacLir!
Please lift the veil so the Goddesses and Gods
May join with us here.
Part aside the watery veils,
Between us and the Spirit realms,
Sail them, to our earthly shore,
To join with us once more.
O Manannán! Lord of the Headlands and Son of the Sea,
May the Gods and Spirits mingle with us freely!

Call in the Three Worlds of the Ancestors, Nature Spirits, and Gods

We now invoke the sacred three: Land, Sea, and Sky!
Ancestors in the sacred land, you whose blood and bone have made
the soil upon which we stand,
You whose sacrifice of laughter and tears have enabled us to be
alive today,
You whose teachings and Spirit have been bequeathed to us in our
books and traditions and in our listening,
We honor you and we welcome you into our circle!

Nature Spirits, seen and unseen,
You who have given your flesh, blood, and fur
so that we may eat and live,
You who have given us your love,
We welcome you here, winged, scaley, furred, and feathered ones!
Also, the trees and herbs of the forests and fields,
The mighty Sidhe beneath the hills,
And the Elementals who make our gardens grow,

Please be with us in our circle. We thank you and we honor your
presence here!

All the Gods and Goddesses of our people, known and unknown,
named and unnamed,
You of the Sky Realms,
You whose wisdom and care have guided us through all the seasons
of our lives,
Be with us here in our circle!
We honor you and ask for your blessings!

Call in the Sacred Five Directions

Wise Salmon of the East! Bringer of abundance!
Welcome to our circle.
Please bestow upon us prosperity, fat cattle,
and hives rich with honey.
May we all have beautiful raiment, warm firesides,
and delicious food!
Keeper of the realm of Earth, bless us with fertility and wealth.
Welcome sacred Salmon!

Great Sow of the South!
You who delve deep into the darkest spaces to bring up
truth and inspiration,
Please bless us with your presence! Bring us your gifts
of poetry, song, and music.
We honor you and your creativity.
From the deep realms of sacred Water,
we welcome you to our circle.
Be with us now!

Sacred Stag of the West!
Guardian of air and of history, storytelling and genealogy,
Please be with us in this sacred space!
We honor your wisdom and determination.
Show us a good direction.
Help us persevere in our learning, teaching, and study.

Great Stag, please be with us now!

Fire Eagle of the North!
Keeper of the Sword of Light and Great Lord of Battle,
Defender of the realms, please be with us now.
Teach us to be fearless. Teach us to protect the ancient
ways of the tribes.
Help us to be a shield for the people!
Great Eagle from the realm of sacred Fire, be with us now!

Great Mare of Sovereignty!
You who stand in the center of all that is, seeing all,
from every direction,
Please be with us here in our circle.
Teach us self-mastery and keep us centered on our path.
Help us do what is right for all lives!
We welcome you here. Be with us now!

Honor An Cailleach

An Cailleach,
Bone Mother,
Queen of Winter,
Shaper of the Lands,
Gnarled One,
Hidden One,
Goddess of Sovereignty,
Deer Mother,
Traveler with Wolves,
Wise Counselor,
Reaper of Lives,
Ancient Hag,
Dark Mother,
Ageless Shadow upon the Hills,
Your children are tired.
Your children are cold.
Your children are hungry.
Spread your soft, snow-filled blanket.

Upon them.

Let there be rest.

Let there be comfort.

Let there be a healing

And rebirth

For the tribes,

For the nations.

Let them be purified,

Let them be renewed,

Let them be safe,

Under your keeping.

Petition for Healing

There comes a time in every person's life when they embark on an
Underworld journey.

We will all visit the Underworld more than once during the course
of our lives.

This journey may begin with the loss of a loved one, or a life-
threatening illness, or a grave disappointment in our career or craft.

When this happens, we feel lost and adrift and separated from
everything we once held dear.

Everything we once knew, our certainty, is gone, and we are set adrift.

We are in shock. We despair. We grieve.

Then we descend to the realm of the Old One, the Crone, the
Cailleach, Lady Death, Hecate, Baba Yaga, Ereshkigal, La Santa
Muerte: She who bears a thousand names.

She hears us. She understands. We have but to ask.

Make now your petitions to her for healing!

[Everyone speaks their need now, separately or together, out loud or silently.]

Know that the ancient Goddess of the Land has heard your petition!

Petition for Future Projects and Visions

Here is the place to dream in your future in the coming season.

Make now your petition for future blessings!

[Everyone speaks their vision, separately or together, out loud or silently.]

Divination

A Seer now seeks the will of the Gods by performing a divination. They may be looking for a message that the ritual has been accepted by the Gods and Goddesses, or they may search for a message that benefits the group as a whole. They may use tarot cards or another deck, bones, stones, ogham sticks, or any other method they are comfortable with.

If the omens are good, the rite can close down. If the omens are bad, another ritual may need to be performed or another divination done to clarify the message.

Close the Rite

The Gods have spoken!

Wise Salmon of the East!
Thank you for gracing us with your presence here.
May your journey throughout the seas be swift and sure.
Hail and farewell!

Great Sow of the South!
Thank you for your gifts to us of music and song.
Long may you delve the dark places to bring forth creativity!
Hail and farewell!

Mighty Stag of the West!
Thank you for keeping our learning alive.
Thank you for inspiring our knowledge.
Hail and farewell!

Fire Eagle of the North!
Thank you for giving us determination and certitude.
Thank you for your strength!
Hail and farewell!

Sacred Mare of Sovereignty!
Thank you for keeping us centered, like the mighty Oak.
Thank you for making us kings and queens within our own realms.
Thank you for the gift of mastery.
Hail and farewell!

Great Hag of Winter!
Bone Mother,
Keeper of the deer,
Rider upon wolves,
Creatrix of the lands,
We see your beauty everywhere—in the winter snows, in the frozen
ice, in the wind-bent trees.
Thank you for your gifts of peace and purification in this season
of winter.
Hail and farewell!

Thank you to all the Gods and Goddesses of our people,
The known and the unknown,
You who have guided and protected us through the generations!
Thank you for your presence here.
Hail and farewell!

We send thanks to the Three Worlds!
To the Sacred Land and to the Realms of Sea and Sky!
Thank you for giving us a place to dwell within the universes.
Hail and farewell!

All thanks to the Nature Spirits!
The furry, finny, scaley, creepy, crawly, and winged ones.
Thank you for feeding us, for your beauty, for your love.
Hail and farewell!

Thank you, ancestors!
For being with us once again in our circle,
For your ceaseless faith, toil, and care,
And the wisdom and determination to survive so we could all be
here today.
Hail and farewell!

O God of the Headlands and Son of the Sea,
Great Manannán MacLir, we thank you for your help here today!
Please close the veil so that only the good may remain,
Only the highest and best for all the people.

O Manannán, please close the portal
And sail us safely home!

Sharing of Cakes and Wine

Serpents are ancient symbols of wisdom because they delve deep into the Earth and bring back her secrets. They are also emblems of healing and trans-formation because they know how to shed their skin and re-create themselves. The reverence for snakes and serpents is seen in many cultures; for example, the ancient Greek caduceus, a symbol of the healer's art, features two twined snakes, while the ancient Picts carved snakes onto their boundary stones.

At the start of the new solar cycle, it is traditional in many cultures to share a snake cake (see one recipe below). When your ritual is closed, bring out the cake on a large tray, covered with bright red cloth and fresh winter greenery. Wassail, spiced cider, mulled wine, eggnog, or any other seasonal beverage should be served with the cake.

When everyone has eaten, say:

Thus ends our rite!
Thank you all for your presence here.
Safe travels and safe home!
Until the wheel turns once more
And we meet again!

🐍 Snake Cake

Snake cakes for the Winter Solstice Season are a tradition found in many cultures, including those of Algeria, Morocco, Greece, Spain, Turkey, Bulgaria, and Italy, just to name a few. The cakes are shaped to look like a coiled snake and are decorated with pine nuts, candied cherries, almonds, and other foods that can be arranged to look like scales or eyes.

Small tokens can be baked inside the cake as a kind of New Year's divination: coins for wealth and luck, a ring for marriage, a bean or pea for not marrying this year, a tiny bit of rag for poverty, a stick for an unhappy marriage, a small religious icon to show a spiritual vocation, and so on.

Adapted from Rosella Rago's "Christmas Torciglione from Umbria," Cooking with Nonna (website), accessed December 28, 2020.

There should be enough pieces so everyone has a slice, and one left over for the household Fairies.

Here is one such recipe, an Italian torciglione *from Umbria.*

> 3 free-range organic egg whites
> 1 pound almonds, ground
> 4 tablespoons ground bitter almonds, ground hazelnuts,
>   or ground walnuts
> 1¼ cups organic sugar or ¾ cup raw, local honey
> 2 tablespoons brandy
> $^{1}/_{3}$ cup organic all-purpose flour (wheat or gluten-free),
>   plus extra for dusting the work surface
> 1 free-range organic egg yolk, lightly beaten
> Whole almonds or pine nuts, for the scales
> 2 whole organic coffee beans or organic candied cherries,
>   for the eyes

Preheat the oven to 350°F and prepare a lightly greased or parchment lined baking sheet.

In a large bowl, beat the egg whites until they form soft peaks. Add the ground almonds, ground bitter almonds, sugar, brandy, and flour and mix well to make a dough.

Roll the dough on a floured work surface, shaping it to make a long stick about 1½ inches thick. If you're using divinatory tokens, poke them into the dough now.

Mold one end of the dough into a pointed "tail" and the other end into a "head." Brush the whole length of dough with the beaten egg yolk. Arrange almonds or pine nuts all over the cake to make "scales." Place the coffee beans or candied cherries in the head to make "eyes." Put one almond or pine nut in the "mouth" to make a tongue.

Curl the snake on the baking sheet. Bake for 30 minutes.

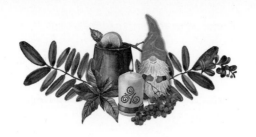

CHRISTMAS TRADITIONS AND RECIPES FROM AROUND THE WORLD

This is just a small sampling of customs and foods of the Yuletide season from around the world. While not an exhaustive list, it should provide inspiration for your own holiday festivities. Some of these foods and activities are modern inventions, while others go back to ancient Pagan times, such as, for example, the custom of inserting a small object into a festive cake as a type of seasonal divination. Why not try introducing some of these seasonal pursuits and recipes into your own family celebration?

Australia (and Britain)

Australians, following British tradition, celebrate with a Christmas tree, a wreath on the door, presents left under the tree, and lights. They have school pageants and caroling, and they leave out food and water for Father Christmas and the kangaroos that pull his sled across the sky. Due to the hot weather, Christmas is a good excuse for a day at the beach.

Even though it is high summer and often quite hot, the Aussie Christmas dinner seeks to emulate traditional British fare. It often features turkey, roast beef, or ham, with mashed Potatoes, gravy, Cranberry sauce, and vegetables. But some families do bow to the hot weather, serving salads, cold meats, and seafood.

For dessert, Pumpkin or Apple pie, Raisin pudding, Christmas pudding, or fruitcake might be on offer. Christmas pudding or Plum pudding is a round, boiled dessert that is properly served flaming with brandy and garnished with a sprig of Holly. A divinatory item—a ring, coin, button, or thimble—might be hidden inside the pudding to divine one's luck in the coming year.[1]

⤚ Traditional British Christmas Pudding

For best results, make the pudding in November and serve it at Yule. You'll need a steamer basket big enough to hold the pudding.

Traditionally, a silver coin is hidden inside the Christmas pudding. The silver coin brings good fortune to whoever is lucky enough to find it when the pudding is cut. But these days real silver coins are no longer in circulation (unless you have an antique one on hand). You can also hide a single almond in the pudding for luck.

Makes 8 servings

    Organic butter, for buttering the basin or bowl

    3¼ cups finely chopped dried organic fruits of mixed varieties

    2 tablespoons finely chopped candied organic citrus peels (see below for instructions on making your own)

    1 small organic apple, peeled, cored, and finely chopped

    2 tablespoons organic orange juice

    1 tablespoon organic lemon juice

    ¼ cup brandy, plus a little extra for soaking at the end

    7½ tablespoons organic self-rising flour (wheat or gluten-free)

    1½ teaspoons ground cinnamon

    1 teaspoon pumpkin pie spice (or mixed spice—British)

    1 scant cup suet (beef or vegetarian), shredded

    7¼ tablespoons organic dark brown sugar

Adapted from Elaine Lemm's "British Christmas Pudding," The Spruce Eats (website), accessed January 2, 2020).

1 tablespoon grated organic orange zest

1½ teaspoons grated organic lemon zest

1 cup fresh organic breadcrumbs

1½ generous cups whole almonds, roughly chopped

2 free-range organic eggs

For Serving

A few tablespoons of brandy, rum, or whiskey, warmed

Hard sauce (such as brandy butter or rum butter)

Organic cream or lemon cream (optional)

Organic ice cream, custard, or sweetened béchamel
 (optional)

Lightly butter a 5-cup pudding basin or a heatproof glass bowl that will fit in your steamer.

Place the dried fruits, candied peels, chopped apple, and orange and lemon juices in a large mixing bowl. Add the brandy and stir well. Cover the bowl with a clean towel and let marinate for a couple of hours, and preferably overnight.

When you're ready to proceed, set a pot of water big enough to hold your steamer on the stove. Heat to a simmer, and keep it hot.

While the water is heating, combine the flour, cinnamon, and pumpkin pie spice in a very large bowl and mix well. Add the suet, sugar, orange and lemon zests, breadcrumbs, and almonds and mix well. Add the marinated fruit mixture and stir again. Press the genuine silver coin or almond into the mix. Beat the eggs lightly in a small bowl, then stir them quickly into the dry ingredients. The mixture should have a fairly soft consistency.

Spoon the mixture into the greased pudding basin, gently pressing it down with the back of a spoon. Cover with a double layer of parchment paper, then a layer of aluminum foil. Tie securely with string, wrapping the string around the basin, then looping over the top and around the bowl again to form a handle, which will be useful when removing the pudding from the steamer.

Place the pudding in a steamer set over the pot of simmering water and steam the pudding for 7 hours. Check the water level frequently so it never boils dry.

The pudding should be a dark brown color when fully cooked. Remove the pudding from the steamer and let cool completely.

Remove the paper, prick the pudding with a skewer, and pour in a little extra brandy. Cover it with fresh parchment paper and retie with string.

The pudding cannot be eaten immediately; it needs to be stored in a cool, dry place and rested, then reheated on Christmas Day. Eating the pudding immediately after cooking will cause it to collapse, and the flavors will not have had time to mature.

On Christmas Day, reheat the pudding by steaming it again for about an hour. Dress the pudding with 2 to 3 tablespoons of warmed brandy, rum, or whiskey and set it alight (turn off the lights in the room so people can see the flames). Then pour on hard sauce (usually brandy butter or rum butter), cream, or lemon cream, or pair with ice cream, custard, or sweetened béchamel.

Leftover Christmas pudding can be refrigerated or frozen (well wrapped) and then reheated by wrapping it tightly in aluminum foil and heating it in a hot oven.

Candied Citrus Peels

Place chopped or sliced lemon and orange peels in a saucepan and barely cover them with water. Boil for 20 minutes, then drain. In a separate saucepan, mix 2 cups organic cane sugar and 1 cup water. Bring to a boil and cook until a small amount dropped in cold water forms a soft thread. Stir in the peels and simmer for 5 minutes, stirring frequently. Drain. Roll the peels, a few pieces at a time, in organic cane sugar. Let them dry on a wire rack for several hours and then store in an airtight container. The peels can then be eaten as candy or added to baked goods and other recipes.

Austria

On December 6, Saint Nicholas's Day, children place shoes by the window so the saint will fill them with sweets when he passes by. Shaggy, horned Krampus figures appear in the streets, frightening onlookers with their noise and devilish appearance. The twelve days of Christmas are said to be rife with demonic activity, so masked figures with brooms parade around town to "sweep away" evil influences. Homes are purified by smoke. On Christmas Eve, the Christ Child brings presents and the Christmas tree is illuminated with real candles.

Traditional fare includes *Vanillekipferl* (Vanilla crescent-shaped cookies), *Zimtsterne* (Cinnamon star cookies), *Sachertorte* (dry, glazed chocolate cake, often filled with Apricot jam), and *Linzertorte* (a rich pastry with a bottom crust and lattice top made of a spiced ground-Almond dough and a filling of Raspberry jam), with *Sektwein* (sparkling wine) or *Gluhwein* (mulled wine) as beverages.

Zelten—butter-yeast dough pies with varied fillings, such as Poppy or Apple—are also served. In the Tyrol region, they are made with dried fruits. If a man wants to marry a woman, he will follow her and offer to carry her *zelten* as she walks to visit her relations. If she says yes, the engagement is on.

Lebkuchen are a bar-type cookie made with Ginger that are often hung on the Christmas tree. If you're making them yourself (see the recipe below), you can bake the cookies with a small hole at the top through which you can pull a red, gold, or green silk ribbon for hanging them.

🌀 Lebkuchen

Makes 40 cookies

For the Dough
7 tablespoons raw, local honey

¾ cup organic brown sugar

4 tablespoons organic butter

2¾ cups organic all-purpose flour (wheat or gluten-free),
   plus more for dusting the work surface

1½ teaspoons aluminum-free baking powder

1 free-range organic egg yolk

1 cup walnuts, ground

5 teaspoons Lebkuchen spice blend, store-bought or
   homemade (see below)

2 teaspoons ground cinnamon

Pinch of grated organic lemon zest

Adapted from Helene Dsouza's "Classic Lebkuchen Cookies Recipe," Masala Herb (website), December 6, 2017.

For Decoration

Chopped candied fruits, such as cherries, ginger, and
orange or lemon peel (optional)

Chopped nuts, such as walnuts, almonds, pistachios,
hazelnuts, and pecans (optional)

Royal icing (optional; see recipe on page 177)

Molded sugar decorations (optional)

Place the honey, brown sugar, and butter into a double boiler and as the
butter melts, mix to a smooth, sticky paste. Put the paste into a bowl and add
the flour and baking powder, then make a well in the center to add the egg
yolk. Add the ground walnuts, Lebkuchen spice mix, cinnamon, and lemon
zest. Mix with a wooden spoon and then keep stirring for 10 minutes to make
a smooth dough.

Preheat your oven to 350°F and prepare a lightly greased or parchment
lined baking sheet.

Turn out the dough onto a floured work surface. Roll it out to about ¼ inch
thickness (don't roll it out too thin!).

Dust the top of the rolled-out dough with flour to prevent sticking.
Use cookie cutters to cut out shapes, or cut them by hand. Then transfer
the cookies to the baking sheet. If you're using nuts and candied fruits for
decoration, press them lightly into the dough.

Bake smaller Lebkuchen cookies for about 15 minutes and bigger ones for
20 minutes. Then remove them from the oven and transfer to a wire rack to cool.

Once the cookies have cooled, you can decorate them with the icing and
top them with colorful sugar decorations, if desired. Either pipe thin lines of
icing onto the cookies or coat their entire surface with a thin layer of icing.

Store the Lebkuchen in a sealed container between layers of parchment
paper. They'll keep for a couple of weeks. If ambient conditions are very dry,
put some apple peels in the container to keep the moisture in the cookies.

Make Your Own Lebkuchen Spice Mix

*Use this mix to make Lebkuchen cookies. If you have any left over, you can also
use it on cinnamon rolls, apple pie, and pumpkin pie.*

5 tablespoons ground cinnamon

1½ tablespoons ground cloves

1 teaspoon ground allspice

1 teaspoon ground cardamom

1 teaspoon ground ginger

1 teaspoon ground mace or nutmeg

¾ teaspoon ground aniseed

France

French children open their Advent calendars in the month of December, as they do in many other regions. They also write letters to Père Noël (Father Christmas), and by French law they must receive a postcard response. A *crèche* (Nativity scene) might be assembled in the home, which stays up until February 2. The children leave shoes by the fireplace in hopes that Father Christmas will fill them with presents.

A Cherry Yule Log is often burned in the fireplace; the log is carried into the home on Christmas Eve and sprinkled with red wine to make it smell extra nice when lit. The log and candles are left burning all night, with some food and drink set aside, just in case Mary and baby Jesus come by during the night.

At midnight on Christmas Eve, the feasting begins. The fare can include roast turkey with Chestnuts or roast goose, oysters, foie gras, lobster, venison, and cheeses. A chocolate sponge cake log called a *bûche de Noël* (Yule Log) is normally eaten for dessert, and in some parts of France, thirteen different desserts are served!

On January 6, Three Kings' Day, French families may enjoy a Galette des Rois (King's Cake), a flat Almond cake decorated with a golden paper crown. A small porcelain object, called a *fève*, is hidden inside the cake, and the person who finds it in their serving is proclaimed the king or queen for the day, wears a pretend crown, and can choose their own king or queen.[2]

🔥 Flourless Buche de Noel (Yule Log Cake)

Makes about 12 servings

For the Filling
2 cups organic heavy cream
½ cup organic confectioners' (powdered) sugar
½ cup unsweetened cocoa powder
1 teaspoon pure vanilla extract

For the Cake
6 free-range organic egg yolks
¾ cup organic sugar
$1/3$ cup unsweetened cocoa powder
1½ teaspoons pure vanilla extract
$1/8$ teaspoon sea salt
6 free-range organic egg whites
Organic confectioners' (powdered) sugar, for dusting
Slivered almonds, for decoration (optional)
Sprig of pine and/or pine cones, for decoration (optional)

Make the Filling

In a large bowl, whip the cream, confectioners' sugar, cocoa powder, and vanilla until the mixture is thick and stiff. Refrigerate the whipped cream until you're ready to use it.

Make the Cake

Preheat the oven to 375°F. Line a jelly roll pan with parchment paper. (A jelly roll pan, typically measuring 10½ by 15½ inches, is a smaller version of a rimmed baking sheet.)

In a large bowl, beat the egg yolks with ½ cup sugar until thick and pale. Blend in the cocoa powder, vanilla, and salt.

In a separate large bowl, using clean beaters, whip the egg whites into soft peaks. Gradually add the remaining ¼ cup sugar, beating until the whites form stiff peaks. Immediately fold the yolk mixture into the whites.

Adapted from Tyrarachelle's "Buche de Noel," Allrecipes (website), accessed January 17, 2021.

Spread the batter evenly in the prepared pan. Bake for 12 to 15 minutes, until the cake springs back when lightly touched.

Lay a clean dishtowel on your work surface and dust it with confectioners' sugar. Run a knife around the edge of the pan to free the cake, then turn the warm cake out onto the towel. Remove and discard the parchment paper.

Starting at the short edge of the cake, roll the cake up with the towel. Let cool for 30 minutes.

Unroll the cake. Spread the whipped-cream filling to within 1 inch of the edge. Roll the cake up again, with the filling inside. Place seam-side down on a serving plate and refrigerate until serving.

Dust with confectioners' sugar right before serving, to resemble snow. Add slivered almonds, if you like, to mimic bark. A sprig of pine and a few pine cones on the side of the dish make a nice woodsy touch, too. When finished, the cake should look like a tiny Yule Log.

French Canada

Christmas Eve is the time for the traditional Québécois *réveillon,* a nightlong dinner and dance party. The word comes from the verb *réveiller,* "to wake up." People may even sleep during the day to be ready to frolic on Christmas Eve.

The réveillon is the biggest feast of the year and may feature *tourtière* (meat pie), *ragoût de patte* (pig's feet stew), turkey with all the trimmings, vegetables, ham, pea soup, Maple syrup, and more. There is likely also a *bûche de Noël* for dessert.

The réveillon may be held before, instead of, or after midnight Mass. The feast is usually followed by dancing and the exchange of gifts. Santa Claus might even drop by for a visit to distribute presents. Christmas morning is when presents are opened, followed by a day of visiting with family and friends, ending with a huge dinner.[3]

🥟 Tourtière (Meat Pie)

You can make this ahead of time and freeze it for later. If you don't want to bother with making your own pastry, buy premade pastry shells at the supermarket.

Makes 8 servings

For the Pastry

2 cups unbleached organic all-purpose flour (wheat or gluten-free)

½ teaspoon kosher salt

²/₃ cup organic butter or lard

6–7 tablespoons cold water

For the Filling

2 large organic potatoes, peeled and cut into 2-inch chunks

1 pound organic ground beef

1 pound organic ground pork

1 small organic onion, finely chopped

1 clove organic garlic, finely minced

½ teaspoon poultry seasoning

½ teaspoon ground cinnamon

¼ teaspoon ground cloves

¼ teaspoon ground nutmeg

¼ teaspoon kosher salt

¹/₈ teaspoon freshly ground black pepper

1 free-range organic egg, lightly beaten

Make the Pastry

Combine the flour with the salt in a large bowl. Cut in the butter or lard until the mixture has a roughly even, sandy, crumbly texture. Add the water and blend just until the dough comes together. Shape the dough into a rough ball, wrap it in plastic, and chill in the refrigerator. While the pastry is chilling, prepare the filling.

Adapted from Rachel Arsenault's "Tourtière: A French-Canadian Meat Pie Recipe," *Grow a Good Life* (website), December 14, 2015.

Make the Filling

Boil the potatoes in a pot of water until tender, about 12 minutes. Reserve ½ cup of the potato cooking water and drain the rest. Mash the potatoes and set aside.

In a large skillet, cook the beef, pork, onion, and garlic over medium heat until no longer pink. Drain off excess fat.

Combine the poultry seasoning, cinnamon, cloves, nutmeg, salt, and pepper in a small bowl, then add the mixture to the meat in the skillet.

Add the reserved potato water to the skillet. Mix well and simmer over low heat for about 10 minutes, until the liquid is absorbed.

Remove the pan from the heat, stir in the mashed potatoes, and set aside to cool.

Assemble and Bake the Pie

Preheat the oven to 400°F.

On a lightly floured surface, divide the dough in half and form each half into a ball. Flatten one ball of dough with your hands, then roll it out to about 12 inches in diameter to fit a 9-inch pie pan. Place the pastry into the pie pan.

Spoon the meat filling into the pie pan. Brush around the outer edge of the pastry with some of the beaten egg.

Roll out the other ball of dough and place it on top of the filling. Fold the top crust under the bottom crust and pinch or flute the edges. Brush the top of the dough with egg wash. Use a sharp knife to cut vent holes.

Bake for 30 to 35 minutes, until the pastry is golden brown. Remove the tourtière from the oven and let cool for at least 10 minutes before serving.

Germany

As in Austria, *Perchten* figures parade through the town, making loud noises while dressed as Demons or as beautiful people, symbolizing the battle between good and evil, darkness and light, winter and spring. The German Perchten parade is an ancient pre-Christian tradition that honors the Goddess Perchta (Berchta, Percht), "The Bright One." Masked figures dance to wake up nature and bring back the light.

On the Rauhnächte (Smoke Nights), from December 21 until January 6, homes are smoked with incense to purify them as guisers shout and make noise in the streets. In the town of Waldkirchen, the Rauhnächt ritual is accompanied by a brass band and men with whips.

On Christmas Eve, a glass pickle is hidden somewhere on the Christmas tree. Good luck and a present come to the one who finds it, usually a child. *Zwetschgenmännla* are "dried fruit people" made from dried Plums, Figs, Raisins, and nuts, with painted Walnuts as heads. Dressed in scraps of cloth, they are good-luck charms for the season. As the saying goes, *Du wirst nie ohne Gold und Glück sein, wenn du einen Pflaumenmenschen in deinem Haus hast* (you will never be without gold and happiness if you have a prune person in your house).

Classic foods at Christmas are roasted goose, rabbit, turkey, or duck, served with Apple and sausage stuffing, dumplings (the classic round ones or one great big loaf-shaped one known as a *Serviettenknödel*), braised Red Cabbage, and stewed Kale, with *Pfeffernuss* cookies spiced with Cinnamon, Allspice, Anise, and Black Pepper and the Christmas bread known as *Stollen* for dessert. Sweet marzipan must be eaten to excess; otherwise, you might be haunted by Demons on Christmas night.

🍂 Stollen

This is my very favorite quick-bread stollen recipe, which I altered slightly to include whole-grain flour, chopped apricots, and lemon zest. I find a hint of lemon makes the bread taste lighter and fruitier.

Makes about a 12 inch long loaf

2½ cups organic whole-wheat flour (or gluten-free substitute)

2 teaspoons aluminum-free baking powder

¾ cup organic sugar (or half as much raw, local honey)

½ teaspoon sea salt

½ teaspoon ground mace

Seeds of 5 or 6 cardamom pods, crushed

¾ cup ground almonds

½ cup organic butter, plus extra melted butter to brush on top

Adapted from Anna Thomas's stollen recipe in *The Vegetarian Epicure* (Vintage Books/ Random House, 1972), 304.

1 cup organic cream cheese, at room temperature

1 free-range organic egg

2 tablespoons brandy

½ teaspoon pure vanilla extract

⅓ teaspoon pure almond extract

½ cup organic currants

½ cup organic golden raisins

¼ cup finely chopped organic dried apricots

¼ cup candied organic lemon peel or 1 heaping
   tablespoon grated organic lemon zest

Organic confectioners' (powdered) sugar

Preheat the oven to 350°F.

Sift the flour with the baking powder, sugar, salt, mace, and cardamom seeds into a medium bowl. Stir in the ground almonds. Cut in the butter with a pastry blender or in a food processor until the texture is like coarse sand.

In a separate large bowl, cream the cream cheese, egg, brandy, vanilla, and almond extract. Mix in the currants, raisins, apricots, and candied lemon peel. Add the flour mixture and stir until well blended. Knead the dough into a ball.

Set the ball of dough on a floured work surface. Knead for a few minutes, until smooth.

Shape the loaf into an oval and then crease the loaf down the middle with a knife, off to one side, lengthwise. Fold the smaller side over the larger side to make a 10-inch-long oval (about 8 inches wide in the middle).

Place the loaf on an ungreased baking sheet. Brush lightly with melted butter. Bake for 45 minutes.

Let cool, then dust with organic confectioners' sugar (using a kitchen sieve and knocking the sugar evenly through it to coat the loaf).

Greece

In this maritime country, boats are often decorated for Christmas, and boats festooned with lights even appear in the town squares. Christmas trees were first introduced in the 1800s by King Otto Friedrich Ludwig, who was of Bavarian origin. Now Greeks decorate Fir trees in their homes and in the squares of rural towns.

On the mornings of Christmas Eve and New Year's Eve, children may go from house to house singing carols. The lyrics wish luck and prosperity on the families. While singing, the children play little metal triangles and drums.

The Greek Santa Claus is Aghios Vasilis, meaning Saint Basil. He is the one who brings gifts to children on New Year's Eve. A special cake dedicated to Saint Basil is served after midnight on New Year's Eve and traditionally has a golden coin hidden inside. The cake is divided into sections before serving: one for each family member, one for the saint, and one for the poor. The person who finds the coin in their piece is considered lucky for all the coming year, but if the coin is found in the section dedicated to the poor, it is given away as charity.

On Epiphany Day (January 6), the village priest goes from home to home around the village and sprinkles blessed water into the rooms of the houses so that any hobgoblins go back down to the Underworld.

Pomegranates have been a symbol of good luck, youth, and fertility since ancient times. In many Greek villages on New Year's Day, the house-holder stands outside the front door and breaks open a Pomegranate by hitting it hard on the floor so that the seeds spread everywhere and bring happiness, good health, and abundance to the family.[4]

Traditional foods for the Christmas meal include *avgolemono* (egg, Lemon, chicken, and Rice soup), *lahanodolmades* (Cabbage dol-mades) or *lahanophylla yemista* (stuffed Cabbage leaves), *christopsomo* bread, *kouloures* (basically Greek bagels), pork stew, *melomakarona* and *kourabiethes* cookies, *loukoumades* (honey dough balls), *karidopita* (Walnut spice cake), *kalitsounia kritis* (cheese pastries), and baklava.

🍲 Greek Karidopita (Walnut Cake)

Makes about 15 servings

For the Cake

7 free-range organic eggs
1 cup organic vegetable oil

Adapted from Lynn Livanos Athan's "Karidopita: Greek Walnut Cake," The Spruce Eats (website), accessed January 24, 2021.

½ cup organic milk (or nondairy substitute)

2 cups organic sugar

2 tablespoons brandy or cognac

Zest of 1 organic lemon

2 teaspoons ground cinnamon

$\frac{1}{8}$ teaspoon ground cloves

3½ cups organic self-rising flour (wheat or gluten-free)

2 teaspoon aluminum-free baking powder

1 teaspoon baking soda

1 cup walnuts, coarsely ground

A few walnuts, chopped, for topping

For the Syrup

2 cups organic sugar

2½ cups water

1 small piece cinnamon stick

Juice of ½ organic lemon, strained

Make the Cake

Preheat the oven to 350°F. Grease and flour a 9- by 12-inch baking pan or a similarly sized round pan. (You can also line the bottom of the pan with parchment to make it easier to remove the cake.)

In a large bowl, beat the eggs until they are a light-yellow color, about 5 minutes. Add the oil, milk, and sugar and mix well. Add the brandy, lemon zest, cinnamon, and cloves and mix briefly.

In a separate bowl, sift the flour with the baking powder and baking soda. Slowly mix the flour mixture into the batter. Stir in the ground walnuts.

Pour the cake batter into the prepared baking pan and bake for 35 to 40 minutes, until a knife inserted into the center of the cake comes out dry.

While the cake is baking, prepare the syrup.

Make the Syrup

Combine the sugar, water, and cinnamon stick in a small saucepan and bring to a low boil. Simmer, uncovered, for about 10 minutes, until the syrup thickens slightly. Remove from the heat, remove the cinnamon stick, and stir in the lemon juice. Allow the syrup to cool to room temperature.

Assembly

Remove the cake from the oven. Pour the cooled syrup over the warm cake. Top with a few chopped walnuts as decoration.

Iceland

Iceland is an unusually literate, book-loving society, and on Christmas Eve, Icelanders exchange books as gifts and then spend the night reading them, often while drinking hot chocolate or an alcohol-free Christmas ale called *jólabland*.

Cemeteries are often decorated with lights over the Christmas season. Instead of Santa Claus or Father Christmas, children are visited by the thirteen Yule Lads (see page 24). Christmas dinner usually includes roast lamb (in the old days the lamb was smoked over sheep's dung!). There may also be *humarsúpa* (langoustine soup), *jólarjúpa með berjasósu* (grouse with berry sauce), smoked salmon, herring, turkey, goose, ptarmigan, reindeer, *kryddað rauðkál með bláberjum* (Cabbage with Blueberries), *brúnaðar kartöflur* (glazed Potatoes), rye bread, *laufabraud* ("leaf bread," meaning thin cakes cut into intricate designs and fried in oil), *vínarterta* (Prune jam layer cake), and *jolagrautur* (Rice pudding).

🌱 Kryddað Rauðkál með Bláberjum (Spiced Cabbage with Blueberries)

This traditional Christmas side dish pairs well with grouse, ham, beef, and lamb.

Makes 6–8 servings

> 2 tablespoons organic unsalted butter
>
> 1 medium organic red onion, thinly sliced
>
> 2 cups fresh organic blueberries
>
> ½ cup organic red currant jam
>
> ¼ cup red wine vinegar
>
> 2 teaspoons ground cinnamon

Adapted from Nanna Rögnvaldardóttir's "Spiced Cabbage with Blueberries (Kryddað Rauðkál með Bláberjum)," reproduced on the *Saveur* website from its December 2014 issue, accessed January 12, 2021.

1 teaspoon ground ginger

1 large head organic red cabbage, cored and thinly sliced

1 tart organic green apple, such as Granny Smith, cored,
    peeled, and roughly chopped

Kosher salt and freshly ground black pepper, to taste

¼ cup water

Melt the butter in an large saucepan over medium-high heat. Add the onion and cook until soft, 5 to 7 minutes. Add the blueberries, jam, vinegar, cinnamon, ginger, cabbage, apple, salt, pepper, and water. Bring to a boil, then reduce the heat to medium. Cook, covered, until the cabbage is tender, about 1 hour.

Ireland

A traditional Irish Christmas includes placing a light in the window for absent friends, relations, and strangers so they know they are welcome, as well as caroling, processions of Wren Boys (see page 33), attendance at midnight Mass, and perhaps a Christmas Day swim in the sea. The day after Christmas, there are horse races.

The door is decorated with a Holly wreath. Fairy lights, Christmas trees, and other decorations are put up on December 8, the day of the Feast of the Immaculate Conception, and come down on "Little Christmas," or January 6. January 6 is also the day of "Women's Christmas," when the women of a household get to relax and be waited on by others.

On Twelfth Night, January 5 or 6, twelve candles representing the twelve apostles, and sometimes one more to represent Jesus, are lit in the home.

Dinner includes roast turkey, Potatoes, Brussels Sprouts, and various other vegetables. This is followed by mince pies, pudding, and Christmas cake. Chocolates, assorted biscuits, and mulled wine are also popular.

🌱 Irish Christmas Cake

Make this cake a month ahead of time, wrap it in parchment paper and then aluminum foil, and store it in a sealed container. Note that the dried fruits must be soaked in whiskey the night before you get started. If you don't have whiskey, you can use Guinness, stout, or even strong black tea.

Makes about 15 servings

1 cup organic raisins

¾ cup pitted organic dates

¾ cup organic golden raisins

¾ cup quartered organic candied cherries

¾ cup Irish whiskey

16 tablespoons organic butter, plus extra for greasing the pan

13 tablespoons organic sugar

4 free-range organic eggs

1¾ cups organic all-purpose flour (wheat or gluten-free)

2 tablespoons black treacle or molasses

Grated zest of 1 organic lemon

Grated zest of 1 organic orange

1 rounded teaspoon aluminum-free baking powder

½ teaspoon sea salt

1 teaspoon pumpkin pie spice (or mixed spice—British)

¼ teaspoon ground cloves

¼ teaspoon ground ginger

¼ teaspoon grated nutmeg

8 tablespoons ground almonds

The night before making your cake, combine the raisins, dates, golden raisins, and candied cherries in a large bowl. Add ½ cup whiskey, stir well, and let the fruits soak, ideally for about 12 hours.

When you're ready to bake, preheat the oven to 300°F. Set a rack in the middle of the oven. Butter an 8-inch round cake pan and line it with parchment paper. Wrap some newspaper around the outside of the pan and

---

Adapted from Zack Gallagher's "Traditional Irish Christmas Cake Recipe the Whole Family Will Enjoy," *Irish Central* (website), November 30, 2021.

secure it with string. This wrapping will help keep the outside of the cake from browning too much during the cooking and prevent it from drying out.

In a large bowl, beat together the butter and sugar until creamy. Add the eggs one at a time, dusting a little of the flour into the bowl with each egg added. Add the treacle and grated lemon and orange zest and mix well.

Sift the flour and baking powder into the bowl of soaked fruit, then add the salt, spices, and almonds. Stir all of this together, mixing well. Then fold this fruit mix into the egg mix, stirring evenly.

Spoon the batter into the prepared cake pan. Bake for 3 hours, then check the cake. If it seems to be browning too much, cover it loosely with aluminum foil. Then cook for another 30 minutes. The cake is done when a knife or skewer inserted into the center comes out clean.

Remove the cake from the oven. Use a skewer to poke small holes all over the warm cake. Spoon the remaining ¼ cup of whiskey over the cake until it has all soaked in. Let the cake cool in the pan.

When the cake is cool, remove it from the pan and peel off the lining paper. Then wrap it anew, first in fresh parchment paper and then in aluminum foil. Set it in a container, cover, and be patient!

Once a week, "feed" the cake: Open the wrappings, pour the brandy, sherry, or whiskey on the top and flip the cake over to pour more on the bottom once a week. Rewrap and put it back into its container. This ensures that all that lovely alcohol penetrates to the very middle of the Christmas cake.

Italy

On December 13, Italians celebrate Santa Lucia. A young girl hands out presents in the saint's name. Children put out their shoes at bedtime so Lucia can fill them with gifts. Babbo Natale, the Italian Santa Claus, appears on Christmas Eve to distribute presents. On January 6, La Befana, the Christmas Witch, comes down the chimney with even more presents—or a lump of coal for naughty children.

Christmas Eve dinner is traditionally a meatless meal featuring many varieties of fish, including *frittura di pesce* (fried fish), such as calamari, baby octopus, or *paranza* (mixed tiny fish). In northern Italy there will be *baccalà* (salt cod), and further south *capitone* (eel). There might also be *accheri ai frutti di mare* (pasta with mixed seafood) a whole roasted fish with Potatoes as a secondo, and then Christmas cookies before midnight Mass.

Christmas dinner might feature *bollito misto* (mixed meats boiled in broth) or a roast, like lamb or *faraona ripena* (guinea fowl stuffed with ground meat and spices), served with *salsa verde* (piquant green sauce) or *mostarda* (candied fruit in spiced syrup). Grilled sausages and chops are also common. Sweet cakelike breads such as *panettone* and *pandoro* are featured desserts.[5]

🌶 Panettone

Yes, panettoni are available now in supermarkets, but those versions are usually loaded with artificial ingredients. Why not make your own?

You will need a bit of special equipment: a stand mixer, an instant-read thermometer, and, ideally, a paper panettone mold, 7 inches wide by 4 inches high. If you don't have a panettone mold, you can also use an oven-safe, straight-sided pot of similar dimensions, a 10-inch cake pan with 2-inch-high sides, or a greased 9-inch tube pan. If you are using a metal pan or pot rather than a paper mold, butter and flour the pan or pot and line them with parchment.

This is a two-day recipe—the dough needs to rise overnight—but well worth the investment of your time.

Makes 12–16 servings

> 5 cups organic all-purpose flour (wheat or gluten-free),
>   plus a little more
> 1 tablespoon instant yeast (slightly more than 1 packet)*
> ⅔ cup lukewarm water
> ½ cup organic dark raisins

Adapted from Sally Vargas's "Panettone," Simply Recipes (website), accessed January 6, 2021.

---

*Note: You can substitute active dry yeast for the instant yeast. If you do, place the water in the bowl first, stir in the yeast, and let stand until bubbly, about 5 minutes. Then stir in the flour. Make sure your yeast is 6 months old or less by checking the date on the packet or container. Old yeast may not rise!

½ cup organic golden raisins

½ cup diced organic candied orange peel or a mixture
   of diced organic dried fruit, such as apricots, pears,
   cranberries, and dried cherries

¼ cup dark rum

¼ cup hot water

½ cup slivered almonds (optional)

1½ teaspoons fine sea salt

5 free-range organic eggs

$^1/_3$ cup organic sugar

2 teaspoons pure vanilla extract

Finely grated zest of 1 organic orange

12 tablespoons (1½ sticks) organic unsalted butter, at
   room temperature, to make the dough

Organic vegetable oil (preferably in a spray canister)

1 tablespoon cold organic unsalted butter, for the top of
   the dough

Day One

In the bowl of a stand mixer, stir together 1 cup of the flour and the yeast. Add the water and mix with a spoon until it has the consistency of thick cake batter. Cover the bowl with plastic wrap and let rise for 45 minutes. The sponge should double in size.

Meanwhile, combine the dark raisins, golden raisins, candied orange peel, rum, and hot water in a small bowl. Cover with a plate. If you're using almonds, measure them out and set the measuring cup on top of the plate (so you don't forget them). Let the fruits soak overnight.

In a medium bowl, whisk together the remaining 4 cups flour and salt until blended.

Once the sponge has risen, transfer it, in its bowl, to a stand mixer fitted with the paddle attachment. With the mixer on medium speed, add the eggs to the sponge one at a time, mixing well after each addition. Then mix in the sugar, vanilla, and orange zest.

Drop the mixer to low speed and gradually add about 2½ cups of the flour mixture. Mix for about 2 minutes, until blended. You may need to scrape down the sides of the bowl. The dough should be very soft and stretchy.

With the mixer still on low speed, gradually add the remaining 1½ cups of the flour mixture, mixing until it is incorporated.

Replace the mixer's paddle attachment with a dough hook if you have one. Use it to knead the dough, on low speed, for about 8 minutes, until the dough is very smooth and elastic. Pause two or three times to push down any dough that creeps up on the dough hook.

With the mixer on low speed, gradually add the butter, a few tablespoons at a time, until it is incorporated. Continue to mix with the dough hook for about 3 minutes, until the dough is silky and shiny. If it still seems extremely sticky, gradually add from 1 to 4 tablespoons of flour. The dough should be very soft and still sticky and will just barely pull away from the sides of the bowl, but not the bottom.

Of course, throughout history cooks have mixed batters and doughs by hand. You can cut in the butter with two knives and mix everything with a wooden spoon until you have a shiny dough!

Keeping the dough in the bowl, pat it into a ball. Spray or brush lightly with vegetable oil, then place a piece of plastic wrap directly on the dough. Let rise in the refrigerator for at least 8 hours and up to 2 days.

Day Two

Place the paper panettone mold on a baking sheet. Drain the fruit.

Turn the dough out onto a floured work surface. With a rolling pin, roll it into a flat rectangle that is approximately 12 inches by 15 inches.

Spread the drained fruit and the almonds evenly over the dough. With the rolling pin, roll forcefully over the fruit and nuts to embed them into the dough.

Imagine that the fruit-covered dough is divided widthwise into thirds— that is, along the 15-inch sides, so that each third is about 5 inches wide. Fold the two outer thirds inward, over the middle third, as if you were folding up a letter. You will end up with a rectangle. Then fold the bottom half of the rectangle up to meet the top, forming a square.

Pat the square to a thickness of about 1½ inches. Then bring the corners in toward the center to form a ball, and pinch the loose ends together. Cup your hands around the dough to round the ball.

Place the dough seam-side down inside the panettone mold. Cover with plastic wrap and let rise in a warm place for 1½ to 2 hours, until the dough reaches the top edge of the mold. (This can take longer if the room is cold.)

About 30 minutes before the panettone is ready to be baked, set a rack in the lower third of the oven. Preheat the oven to 375°F.

When the dough has risen, use a sharp serrated knife to cut a shallow cross from edge to edge across its top, just scoring the surface rather than cutting into it deeply. Place the pat of cold butter in the center of the cross.

Reduce the oven temperature to 325ºF and bake the panettone for 30 minutes. Then place a piece of aluminum foil loosely over the top, to keep it from browning too much, and bake for another 40 to 45 minutes, until the panettone is golden brown and an instant-read thermometer inserted into the center of the dough registers 195°F. (Poke the thermometer in through the side of the cake, through the paper, so you don't mar the top.) Remove the cake from the oven, transfer it to a wire rack, and let cool completely in the paper mold.

Lithuania

At Christmas Eve dinner, straw is placed on the table as a symbol of fertility and the luck of the harvest. An empty place is set for the dead and in honor of distant family members. The meal is meatless and usually features fish such as herring, Potato pancakes, sauerkraut, Beet soup with Mushroom-filled dumplings, vegetable salad, Potatoes, fruits, *kutia, kūčiukai* (small sweet pastries) soaked in Poppy seed milk (cookie soup, basically), *kisielius* (a drink made from Cranberries), *kissel* (a fruit soup/jelly thickened with Potato flour), stewed fruit compote, a Poppy seed roll, and cookies. Food is left on the table after the meal for any wandering Spirits that might happen by.

There is straw under the tablecloth, too, and everyone pulls out a piece. Pulling a long straw means you will have a long life. A short straw means a short life. Unmarried women pull a piece to divine their future mate; pulling a long, thin piece means they will have a tall, thin husband, and a short, thick piece means a short, fat husband. If a married person pulls a thin straw, it means a year of financial hardship, while a thick stalk means a fat wallet. If a married woman pulls a straw that is thick in the middle, it means pregnancy.

Another type of divination is done by dripping hot wax into cold water and examining the shapes it makes. If the wax resembles a type of vehicle, it means a journey. If it looks like a house, a move may be coming. A flower signifies a wedding, a cradle a birth, and a coffin or a candle a death.

The Christmas tree is decorated with straw ornaments, fruit, and candy, and children are shown the tree only after supper. Kaledu Senelis, "Grandfather Christmas," appears in person on Christmas Eve, and each child must "earn" their gift by singing a song, reciting a poem, or playing a musical instrument.[6]

🎵 Lithuanian Aguonų Vyniotinis (Poppy Seed Roll)

Makes about 16 servings

> 2½ cups organic pastry flour (wheat or gluten-free)
> ⅛ teaspoon sea salt
> 1⅓ sticks organic butter, melted, for the dough
> ½ cup water
> 1 free-range organic egg
> 2¾ cups poppy seeds
> ¾ cup organic raisins
> ¼ cup organic sugar
> ½ cup raw, local honey, heated to a thin consistency
> 2 tablespoons organic butter, melted, for basting

Preheat the oven to 325°F. Butter a rimmed baking sheet.

Sift the flour into a large mixing bowl. (If you don't have a sifter, just place a small amount of flour in a sieve and knock the sides, repeating until all the flour has been sieved.) Sprinkle in the salt and then, with your fist, form a well in the center of the flour. Pour in the melted butter, egg (beaten), and water. Mix the ingredients by hand into a smooth dough.

Cover a table with a clean, lint-free tablecloth and set the dough on it. Work the dough with your hands as you would to stretch pizza dough, pulling it

Adapted from Christiana Noyalas's "Lithuanian Poppy Seed Roll Recipe," Lithuanian Music Hall Association (website), accessed January 9, 2021.

outward from the center and from the edges. Continue stretching the dough until it is thin and translucent.

Spread the poppy seeds evenly over the dough to within 1 inch of the edges. Top the poppy seeds with the raisins, sprinkle with the sugar, and drizzle the honey over the seeds and raisins.

Lift one end of the tablecloth so that the dough can be rolled. Carefully continue lifting and rolling until the dough is completely rolled up into the shape of a log.

Place the poppy seed roll on the prepared baking sheet. Bake for 45 minutes. Remove from the oven, baste with half of the remaining melted butter, and bake for 15 more minutes, until golden. Then remove from the oven and baste with the remaining butter.

Let the roll cool, then wrap it tightly with plastic wrap and store in the refrigerator, where it will keep for up to 4 days. Slice and serve.

Mexico

On December 23, called the Noché del Rábano (Night of the Radishes), giant Radishes are carved into the figures from the Nativity. Christmas dinner includes a turkey (a bird that was first domesticated by the Aztecs), chicken, or ham, with tamales, empanadas, posole, Christmas *ponche* (fruit punch), *atole* (a sweet drink), *champurrado* (Mexican hot chocolate), and Rice and Corn pudding. Dessert often features *buñuelos,* a type of deep-fried dough with sugar and spices, such as Cinnamon.

🌢 Mexican Buñuelos

It is probably best to make these crispy, crunchy treats on Christmas Day, or no more than a day or two before.

Makes 8 servings

> 2 cups organic all-purpose flour (wheat or gluten-free)

Adapted from Isabel Orozco-Moore's "Mexican Buñuelos," Isabel Eats (website), December 17, 2018.

1½ teaspoons aluminum-free baking powder
½ teaspoon sea salt
¾ cup warm water
4 tablespoons organic oil, plus 2 or more cups for frying
Organic sugar
Ground cinnamon

Mix together the flour, baking powder, and salt in a large bowl. Add the warm water and 4 tablespoons oil. Using a fork, mix until the dough comes together.

Transfer the dough onto a clean work surface and knead for 8 to 10 minutes, until the dough is smooth and elastic. Roll the dough into a ball, place it in a bowl, cover with a kitchen towel, and let it rest for 30 minutes.

Divide the dough evenly into eight pieces. Roll each piece into a ball. On a lightly floured surface, use a floured rolling pin to roll out each ball into an 8- to 10-inch circle.

Heat the frying oil in a deep pan to 350°F. Lay out a plate with paper towels.

Fry each dough circle for about 60 seconds, turning once with metal tongs, until golden brown on both sides. Transfer to the towel-lined plate to blot excess oil. Garnish with cinnamon sugar and eat!

Note: To minimize very large air pockets, use metal tongs to keep the dough fully submerged in the oil for the first 10 to 15 seconds of frying. This will fry both of the sides at the same time and shorten the cooking time.

Sprinkle the cinnamon sugar on as soon as possible after frying to ensure that it sticks to the dough.

To store, stack the buñuelos on a plate and cover with a paper towel or napkin. They'll keep for up to 3 days. Do not store them in an airtight container or in the fridge, or else they may lose some of their crunchy, crispy texture. Warm them in a low oven for 5 minutes before serving.

Norway

Figures of red-capped Nisser (house Elves), red-and-white-spotted Amanita mushrooms, and red candles are set out as decorations. Julesvenn, the Norse Santa figure, hides Barley stalks around the house, making sure the luck from one year is carried over to the next, thus ensuring a good harvest in the new year.

The eve of December 13 is considered especially dangerous because from that date until Christmas, Spirits, Gnomes, and Trolls are about. The barn door must be marked with a cross to protect it, Spruce is burned in the hearth to keep witches from coming down the chimney, and a Yule Log and Christmas candles must be kept burning all night. Guns are fired to scare away evil Spirits.

On December 13, Saint Lucia's Day, young girls in white dresses with crowns of lights (or candles) on their heads carry candles, cookies, and Saffron buns in procession.

The "Wild Hunt" are said to be active at this time—powerful Spirits who rage across the sky, especially on Solstice night, are said to be active at this time.

In the old tradition of *juleham* (Christmas hay), fresh hay was brought into the main living room on Christmas Eve and spread on the floor. All members of the household, including the servants, gathered together to sleep under one roof for three nights. It was believed that sleeping together and the protective power of the grain kept demonic forces at bay.

At Christmas the *julenek* (a sheaf of Oats) is put out for the birds, and the family Nisse gets a bowl of porridge. Julesvenn asks the children if they have been naughty or nice and then hands out gifts. Children go *julebukk* after Christmas, visiting houses dressed in costumes and receiving treats.

The Christmas dinner features roast pork or spare ribs, *lutefisk* (codfish preserved in lye), *lefse* (Potato flatbread that can be served with butter or sprinkled with Cinnamon and sugar as a dessert), meatballs, *julekake* (Christmas bread with Raisins and candied fruits), and Rice porridge (*risgrøt*) with an Almond hidden inside. According to the custom, whoever gets the Almond wins a prize, will have good luck, or will be married within the year. (Rice porridge is also a feature of Christmas traditions in Denmark. There, it's said that whoever gets the Almond in their bowl will have good luck all year, and they are given a marzipan pig as a prize.)

A "Spirit plate" of food is put out for the departed ancestors.

🍂 Norwegian Risgrøt (Rice Porridge)

Serve this porridge for breakfast, for lunch, or with dinner. You can also leave some out as an offering for Tomte (Gnome-like creatures). If you like, substitute half a vanilla bean for the extract; grind it slightly, add it to the warmed milk, and strain it out when the milk is done.

Makes 4 servings

> ¾ cup organic medium- or long-grain white rice
>
> 1½ cups water
>
> Organic sugar or raw, local honey
>
> Pure vanilla extract
>
> Ground cardamom
>
> 5½ cups organic whole milk
>
> Ground cinnamon, for serving
>
> Organic unsalted butter, for serving
>
> Fresh or frozen berries, for serving

Rinse the rice. Combine the rice and the water in a large saucepan over high heat. Bring to a boil, then reduce the heat and simmer the rice, covered, for about 10 minutes to partially cook it.

Spice and sweeten the rice with the sugar, vanilla, and cardamom to taste.

Stir, and begin adding milk very slowly as you continue to stir. The rice will absorb the milk as you stir it over the heat. Keep stirring for about 40 minutes, continually adding milk just until it is absorbed. Make it a family project, with everyone taking a turn!

When the rice porridge looks creamy and all the milk has been absorbed, it's done! Ladle it into bowls, and serve with a sprinkle of cinnamon, a pat of butter, and some fresh or frozen berries on top.

Adapted from Holly Erickson and Natalie Mortimer's "Norwegian Risgrøt Rice Porridge," The Modern Proper (website), December 19, 2015.

Poland

Presents are given on Mikolajki, (Saint Nicholas's Day), on December 6. Gifts are brought to school and shared with students, and Santa leaves gifts at the house door or under the pillow. More gifts are given on Christmas Eve. Depending on family customs, the gifts may be brought by Gwiazdor (Star Man), Aniolek (Angel), Dzieciatko (Baby Jesus), Śnieżynka (Snowflake), Dziadek Mróz (Jack Frost), or Santa Claus.

The *podlazniczka,* the cut-off top of a Fir, Pine, or Spruce tree, is traditionally hung upside down from the ceiling, usually over the dining room table. It might be ornamented with straw and paper decorations, nuts, fruits (especially Apples, symbolizing good health), candy, gingerbread cookies, crocheted ornaments, and small globular wafers called *światy* (worlds).[7]

Everyone is expected to be on their best behavior on Christmas Eve because it is believed that the way you spend that day is the prediction of your coming year.

Wigilia, sometimes called Wieczerza Wigilijna (Christmas Eve Dinner or Star Supper), begins when the first star appears in the sky. Then the head of the household breaks up the *oplatek* (an unleavened flat wafer made of flour and water) and shares it with the family and guests around the table, from oldest to youngest, wishing good things for each of them in the new year. In the feast that follows, one place is left vacant at the table in case an unexpected wanderer appears, looking for a place to spend Christmas. Hay is put under the table, in memory of Jesus's birth in a manger (and that custom probably goes back to Pagan times, when grain was seen as an agent of fertility and the luck of the harvest).

Pierogis are a traditional dish, made with mashed Potato, fried Onion, and cottage cheese, or with sauerkraut and Mushrooms, or perhaps with dried Plums. *Salatka jarzynowa,* a salad made of Potatoes, pickles, Peas, Carrots, Parsley root, Celery root, and eggs, is also common. There might be Mushroom soup or red borscht served with *uszka* (tiny dumplings filled with dried Mushrooms). A *grosz* (small coin) is hidden inside one of the dumplings, and it's said that the person who finds it will have money throughout the upcoming year.

Other dishes could include *kapusta z grochem* (Cabbage with beans) and carp (fried, cold and jellied in aspic, or baked). There may be cold pickled herring accompanied by eggs, mayonnaise or sour cream, and almost always Onions. Do save the carp fish scales! Some families like to put one scale under each person's plate to bring financial prosperity in the new year. Others keep them in their wallet (and they are a favorite talisman for gamblers).

For dessert there is *kutia* (a traditional Polish Christmas porridge made from Wheat berries; see the recipe on page 53), *kluski z makiem* (a sweet pasta with Poppy seeds and dried fruit and nuts), and *makowiec* (a traditional Polish Poppy seed cake with Raisins).

Kompot z suszu is a Christmas drink made with dried fruits (Apples, Pears, Plums, and Apricots) that are put into a pot with water and sugar and boiled. The drink is served cold.[8]

The Wigilia feast usually features twelve dishes on the table. It is important to taste all twelve because each dish represents one month, and trying every dish guarantees abundant food in the new year. Traditionally, no meat or alcohol is served, and everyone fasts all day in preparation for the feast. After dinner presents are opened, and then it's off to midnight Mass.

The first visitor to cross the threshold on Christmas day scatters grain in the house and the family tosses grain back at them. Then the visitor makes sure to strike the Yule Log so that sparks fly (thus chasing any evil Spirits back up the chimney) and wishes good luck on the family. They might also drop a coin onto the Yule Log for prosperity. They will be invited to stay for dinner and upon leaving are given a gift.[9]

🍲 Kapusta z Grochem (Cabbage with Split Peas)

This dish pairs well with pork or bacon, or serve it as a main dish for your vegetarian friends. It calls for fresh cabbage, but feel free to substitute more sauerkraut, or a mixture of the two.

Makes 6 servings

6 cups water, plus more as needed

1 pound organic dried yellow split peas, rinsed and drained

Adapted from Barbara Rolek's "Split Peas and Cabbage Kapusta z Grochem," The Spruce Eats (website), accessed January 23, 2021.

1 small head organic cabbage, shredded

1 quart sauerkraut, undrained or drained, if desired,
    reserving some of the kraut juice

3 cups water

1 organic onion, finely chopped

2 tablespoons organic butter

Sea salt and freshly ground black pepper, to taste

Bring 3 cups water to a boil in a small saucepan. Add the split peas, bring the water back to a boil, and continue boiling for 2 minutes. Then remove from the heat, cover, and let soak for 30 minutes.

After 30 minutes, bring the pan of peas back to a boil, then reduce the heat and let simmer, covered, for 20 minutes, until the peas are cooked down to a purée, adding more water if necessary. Remove from the heat and set aside.

Meanwhile, in a large pot or Dutch oven, combine the shredded cabbage, sauerkraut, and 3 cups of water. Bring to a boil, then reduce the heat and let simmer, covered, for 1 hour.

While the cabbage is cooking, sauté the onion in the butter until golden brown. Set aside.

When the cabbage is done cooking, stir in the cooked peas. Season to taste with salt and pepper. Add some kraut juice if the mixture seems too dry. Add the sautéed onion and mix well. Heat until warm throughout, then serve.

Russia

Christmas in Russia is celebrated on January 7 because the Russian Orthodox Church uses the Julian calendar.

New Year's is when Ded Moroz (Grandfather Frost) brings presents to children. He has a long white beard and carries a big magic staff as a symbol of his power. He is always accompanied by his granddaughter Snegurochka (Snow Maiden). On New Year's Eve, children hold hands, make a circle around the Christmas tree, and call for Snegurochka or Ded Moroz. When they appear, it's said, the star and other lights on the Christmas tree magically light.

As in Poland, some people fast on Christmas Eve until the first star appears in the sky, and then they eat *sochivo* or *kutia* (Wheat berry or rice porridge; see the recipe on page 53). The porridge may be eaten from one common bowl, symbolizing unity. Some families like to throw a spoonful up on the ceiling; if it sticks to the ceiling, it signifies good luck and a good harvest in the coming year.

Christmas Eve foods include *borscht* (Beet soup) and individual pies made with Cabbage, Potato, or Mushrooms, as well as sauerkraut, porridge dishes such as Buckwheat with fried Onions and fried Mushrooms, potato and other root vegetable salads, and other types of salads, too, often made from vegetables like Gherkins, Mushrooms, or tomatoes. *Vzvar* (meaning "boil up"), a sweet drink made from dried fruit and honey boiled in water, is served at the end of the meal.

The Christmas Day feast features roast pork or goose, *pirog* (a large pie filled with meat and vegetables), and *pelmeni* (meat dumplings). Dessert may be fruit pies, gingerbread, honey cookies (called *pryaniki*), and fresh or dried fruits and nuts. Russian Christmas cookies called *kozulya* are made in the shape of a sheep, goat, or deer.[10]

🍃 Classic Russian Красный Борщ (Red Borscht)

Start with a nice piece of chuck on the bone, plus extra bones, which you can usually get from a butcher, for extra flavor. You can shred all the veggies (except the potatoes and cabbage) in a food processor or hand shredder, or if you have one, a Vitamix—throw everything in, cover with water, and pulse on the "wet chop" setting.

Serve with a dollop of sour cream and warm sourdough bread.

Makes about 6 servings

>   2–3 pounds organic beef chuck roast, on the bone
>   1 pound beef bones
>   2 large organic beets, shredded
>   5 organic carrots, shredded
>   1 large organic onion, shredded
>   3 large (or 6 small) organic yellow potatoes, peeled and
>   cut into chunks

Adapted from Mila Furman's "Classic Russian Borscht Recipe—Красный Борщ," Girl and the Kitchen (website), accessed January 15, 2021.

¾ cup organic tomato puree

Juice of 1 organic lemon

2 tablespoons organic sugar or 1 tablespoon raw, local
     honey

Sea salt and freshly ground black pepper, to taste

Red pepper flakes, to taste

1 small head organic cabbage, shredded

6 cloves organic garlic, minced

3 tablespoons chopped dill

Cut the meat off the roast and into slightly-larger-than-bite-size pieces. Place the meat and bones into a heavy-bottomed large pot. Cover the meat and bones with cold water, leaving about 4 cups of room at the top. Bring up to a boil.

Just before the soup reaches a boil, scum may rise to the surface. Use a slotted spoon to carefully remove any scum, or strain the soup (pour it through a sieve or colander into a large bowl, then pour the clean liquid back into the pot). After straining, return the meat and the bones to the pot as well.

Add the shredded beets, carrots, and onion (with the water from the Vitamix, if you used one) to the soup. Add the potatoes and tomato puree. Add half of the lemon juice, the sugar, salt, pepper, and a nice helping of red pepper flakes. Bring just to a boil, then reduce the heat and let simmer for 15 minutes.

Add the cabbage to the soup, along with the garlic and dill. Let simmer for another 15 minutes.

Once the cabbage is soft, taste the soup for flavor. Add more lemon juice, salt, pepper, sugar, or red pepper flakes as desired. Remove the bones.

This soup actually tastes better the next day. If you decide to serve it the next day, you can remove any extra fat that solidifies on the top after being refrigerated.

Scotland

Until 1560, Christmas was a time of merrymaking in Scotland, with Yule Logs, Abbots of Misrule (the master in charge of Christmas revels, especially in the fifteenth and sixteenth centuries), and parties of social inversion. When dour Protestants took power, Christmas was suppressed as a

"Papist invention" and persons who celebrated "Yuill-day" were punished. Those charged with attending a New Year's party, or with dancing or singing, could even be excommunicated. Bakers who made Yule breads were prosecuted; the church forbade the making of Yule cake or Yule bannock (a large, round cake) into the seventeenth century. Guising, crossdressing, dancing with bells on, and celebrations in the street or home were repressed. Clergy even searched houses for evidence of a Christmas goose or a weaver who had dared to take the day off.

The Highlands and Outer Hebrides escaped these prohibitions and kept practicing Oidche Choinnle (Candle Night)—on Christmas Eve candles were placed in windows to guide the holy family and the wandering dead ancestors to the house; Yule breads and cakes were enjoyed; and dancing, caroling, feasting, and guising continued unabated. In other areas, the old Yule festivities migrated to Hogmanay (New Year's), though the church tried to suppress that, too, without success. Soon, house parties, celebrations in the streets, guisers, and the ringing of bells marked Hogmanay, as well as customs like First Footing (see page 37), saining (purifying the home), and other rituals of purification by fire.

Christmas didn't really catch on again in Scotland until the midtwentieth century, after World War II, partly because the celebration was regarded as an "English" custom. Today, though, Scots celebrate both Christmas and Hogmanay.

Traditional Christmas fare in Scotland includes cock-a-leekie (chicken and Leek) soup as a starter, then roast pork, glazed ham, roast beef, steak pie, or roast leg of lamb, with haggis (a minced mixture of sheep or calf's organs, suet, oatmeal, and seasoning that is boiled in oil or steamed in a bag made from the animal's stomach), followed by black bun (fruit cake covered in pastry), Atholl Brose (a drink made with oatmeal, honey, whiskey, and sometimes cream), Tipsy Laird (a boozy Scottish trifle), a *clootie* dumpling (boiled suet pudding containing dried fruits) with charms hidden inside, or shortbread cookies with coffee or tea.

🍃 Clootie Dumpling

Clootie means "little cloth." Add a bit of chopped apple to the mix to make it softer, if you like, and if you serve it with custard sauce, add a splash of whiskey and a pinch of ginger.

Makes 8 servings

> 4 cups organic self-rising flour (wheat or gluten-free), plus
>   extra for sprinkling the cloth wrapping
> 1¾ cups organic currants
> 1⅔ cups organic raisins
> ¼ pound shredded suet
> 1 cup dry organic breadcrumbs
> 1 cup organic sugar
> 1 free-range organic egg, lightly beaten
> ½ cup organic milk
> 1 tablespoon molasses
> 1 teaspoon aluminum-free baking powder
> 1 teaspoon pumpkin pie spice (or mixed spice—British)
> Pinch of ground ginger (optional)
> Pinch of sea salt
> Cream, ice cream, or custard sauce, for serving

Bring a large pot of water to the boil.

Meanwhile, in a large bowl, combine the flour, currants, raisins, suet, breadcrumbs, and sugar.

In a separate bowl, mix the egg and milk with the molasses, baking powder, pumpkin pie spice, ginger (if using), and salt. Then stir the milk mixture into the flour mixture to form a wet dough.

Dip a heavy, clean cotton cloth in the boiling water, wring it out, and sprinkle it with flour. Place the dough in the center of the cloth, draw the opposite corners together to form a ball, leaving a bit of room for the dumpling to expand, and tie tightly with twine to seal.

Place the dumpling in the boiling water, reduce the heat to hold a low boil, and cook for 3½ hours, topping off the water as needed.

Adapted from Jill Barrett's "Clootie Dumpling," Allrecipes (website), August 22, 2022.

Lift the dumpling from the water, remove the cloth, and dry the dumpling in front of a fire or in a 150°F oven until the surface is no longer wet. Serve warm.

Serve warm with cream, ice cream, or custard sauce.

Tip: You can place a saucer upside down in the pot before you drop in the dumpling. This will prevent your *cloot* or cloth from sticking to the bottom.

Spain

Spanish girls and boys get their presents from the Three Wise Men (Los Reyes Magos), who come on January 6, the day of the Epiphany. But children often get a few presents on Christmas as well. On the day the Reyes come, there's a parade, and the Three Wise Men ride atop floats and throw candy to all.

The Roscón de Reyes (Kings' Cake) is a Christmas staple, made of brioche that is sometimes stuffed with pastry cream and decorated with candied fruits. Its doughnut shape is said to have been inspired by the crowns worn by the Three Wise Men. Hidden inside is a small ceramic toy and sometimes a fava bean; whoever finds the toy in their piece will have luck for the year, but if anyone breaks a tooth on the fava bean, they are supposed to pay for next year's cake.

The same tradition dates back to the Pagan Romans celebrating the Winter Solstice. A similar cake was served at Saturnalia, and the partier who found a hidden treat inside would be dubbed the king of the festival and treated like royalty.

Christmas trees are a recent fashion in Spain, and in many homes you will still find the classic *portal de Belén,* ornate Nativity scenes that also appear in store windows. After the main meal on Christmas Eve, many families head to church for midnight mass.

Catalan families have a unique Christmas tradition: They decorate a wooden log, giving it a face and legs. It's kept in the home or garden and covered with a blanket to keep it from getting cold. The log is called the *caga tió*—the "pooping log." On Christmas Day, children gather around the log and whack it with sticks, singing a song asking the log to poop out candy for them to eat. When the song is finished, they pull back the blanket and find a hoard of candy magically hidden there.[11]

Christmas Eve dinner begins with *entremeses* (appetizers), which may contain sliced ham, chorizo, *morcilla* (black pudding), and cheese. Seafood is often the main course, though turkey is also traditional. Lobster and shrimp are particularly popular, as are a seafood soup or stew. *Cochinillo* (roast suckling pig) is often served, cooked on a bed of Onions and Potatoes. Roast lamb is another favorite. *Escudella* is a Catalan Christmas dish of huge pasta shells, stuffed with mincemeat and floating in meat and vegetable soup.

Turrón (Almond nougat) is a popular Christmas sweet, as are *mantecados* (small sweets made with lard). *Polvorónes* are a type of powdery mantecado that are dusted with confectioners' sugar. *Marzapan* (marzipan) is another popular treat.

Finally, no Spanish Christmas meal is complete without a sparkling glass of cava, the Spanish version of champagne.[12]

🌿 Roscón de Reyes (King's Cake)

Makes about 10 servings

> 4 cups organic all-purpose flour (wheat or gluten-free)
> ½ teaspoon sea salt
> $^1/_3$ cup lukewarm organic milk
> $^1/_3$ cup lukewarm water
> 1 ounce dry baker's yeast
> 6 tablespoons organic butter, at room temperature
> 6 tablespoons organic sugar
> 2 free-range organic eggs
> 1 tablespoon brandy or rum
> Rind of 1 large organic orange, grated
> 1 free-range organic egg white
> 2 cups assorted organic candied fruits, chopped in
>   different sizes

Sift the flour and salt together into a large bowl. Make a well in the middle.

Combine the lukewarm milk and water in a small bowl. Add the yeast and

---

Adapted from David Pope's "Roscón de Reyes Recipe (Spanish Kings' Cake)," *Spanish Sabores* (blog), November 18, 2019.

stir to dissolve, then pour the mixture into the well of the flour. Scrape in just enough flour from around the well to create a thick batter, sprinkle some of the flour on top, and cover with a kitchen towel. Leave the bowl in a warm place for about 15 minutes, until the batter is doughy and sponge-like.

Meanwhile, in a separate medium bowl, beat the butter and sugar until creamy.

Once the dough is appropriately spongy, add to it the eggs, brandy, grated orange rind, and a splash of water. Mix well, until the dough is elastic and a bit sticky. Add the butter and sugar mixture to the dough and mix until smooth.

Shape the dough into a ball and cover in oiled plastic wrap. Keeping it in the large bowl, cover it with a kitchen towel and leave in a warm place, away from drafts, to rise until doubled in size, which will take anywhere 1 to 2 hours, depending on the strength of the yeast culture.

While the dough rises, grease a large baking sheet.

Once the dough has doubled in size, remove the plastic wrap. Punch down the dough and place it on a lightly floured work surface. Knead it for 2 or 3 minutes, and then roll it into a large rectangle, roughly 2 feet by 6 inches. Then roll the dough inward from the long edge to create a sausage shape. Bring the ends together to create the iconic doughnut shape, and place it on the baking sheet.

Want to add the bean or a ceramic toy? Do it now by poking it into the dough.

Wrap the dough with plastic wrap and leave in a warm place to rise until doubled in size, roughly 1 hour.

Preheat the oven to 350°F.

Once the dough has risen, lightly beat the remaining egg white and brush it across the top. Cover the cake in the assorted dried fruits, pushing them in gently so they do not fall off the cake while it is baking.

Bake for 30 minutes, until golden. Let cool on a wire rack before serving.

Sweden

Saint Lucia's Day, on December 13, is a highlight of the Swedish Yuletide celebration.

December 13 was the Winter Solstice, thus, a Pagan festival was turned into the Christian Saint Lucia's Day. According to legend, Lucia, who lived in fourth-century Rome, would secretly bring food to Christians who were hiding in the catacombs under the city. She wore candles on her head so she could see in the dark while keeping her hands free to carry food. She was martyred for her faith in the year 304 CE and was eventually declared a saint. Lucia's name comes from the Latin word *lux* (light), so this celebration echoes the many other light-centered observances of the season, from Advent candles to Christmas tree lights to Hannukah candles and blazing bonfires, hearth fires, and Yule Logs.

In Sweden on Saint Lucia's Day, girls dress in white dresses with a red sash around their waist and a crown of evergreen Lingonberry twigs and candles on their head. As we have seen in other cultures, the evergreens upon their heads are herbs of health and immortality so fittingly the Lucias appear in hospitals and nursing homes, singing a song about Saint Lucia and handing out *pepparkakor* (ginger snap cookies). The Lucias also serve *lussekatts,* buns flavored with Saffron and Raisins, to their parents for breakfast.

In addition to the celebration of Saint Lucia, light is brought to the season through advent candles and lit up stars—a candle is lit each Sunday of Advent and the stars, which may be red or white and made of various materials from straw to paper to wood or metal, commemorate the Christmas Star.

In the Middle Ages, Scandinavians believed that the ancestors returned to their homes during the Christmas season, and therefore the house had to be thoroughly cleaned in their honor. Food and candles were set out on tables, and doors were left open for invisible guests.[13] Beds were left empty for the Spirits of any deceased family members who might come by for a visit.

Christmas Eve day is when the main meal is eaten. At lunch there is a *julbord* (buffet) featuring cold fish, especially herring and salmon. There may be cold meats, cheese, liver pate, salads, pickles, and bread and butter. Warm dishes include meatballs, *prinskorv* (sausages), *kåldolmar* (meat-stuffed cabbage rolls), jellied pigs' feet, *lutfisk* (dried cod served with a thick white sauce), and *revbenspjäll* (oven-roasted pork ribs). Vegetables include Potatoes and Red Cabbage. Sweet pastries and *pepparkakor* are on offer for dessert. *Glogg* (mulled wine) and coffee end the feast. *Risgrynsgröt* (Rice porridge) is served with *hallonsylt* (Raspberry jam) or sprinkled with Cinnamon in the evening after presents have been exchanged.[14] (See the recipe for Norwegian rice porridge on page 92.)

Sweden has a few gift-bringing traditions. As noted above, family and friends generally exchange presents on Christmas Eve. Christmas presents are brought by Jultomte, or Tomte, the Christmas Gnome (the Swedish equivalent of Santa Clause).

The tradition of Secret Santa may have originated from an old Swedish tradition, Julklapp (Christmas knock), where someone knocks on the door of a friend or neighbor and then leaves a small gift, often made of straw or wood. A riddle is included that hints at who left the present.[15]

The Yule Goat is said to oversee Yule celebrations. Between Christmas and New Year, men and children go *julebukking* dressed up as goats and wander from house to house singing and playing pranks. A straw statuette of the Yule Goat is often erected to guard the house and the Christmas tree; straw ornaments festoon the Christmas tree too. Decorating with straw is a celebration of fertility that carries the energy of the Sun and the luck of the harvest from one year to the next.

🌿 Swedish Julskinka (Christmas Ham)

Set out coarse mustard and pickles to accompany the ham.

Makes 10 servings

> 1 (9-pound) boneless, salt-cured, fresh organic ham
> 2 medium organic onions, peeled and chopped
> 1 large organic carrot, peeled and chopped
> 3 quarts water
> 2 bay leaves
> 10 peppercorns

Adapted from "Swedish Christmas Ham (Julskinka)," Kroger (website), accessed January 27, 2021.

10 allspice berries

5 whole cloves

2 free-range organic egg whites

1 tablespoon organic brown sugar

½ cup Swedish mustard

1 cup dry organic breadcrumbs

1 tablespoon coarsely ground black pepper

Preheat the oven to 250°F.

Place the ham in a Dutch oven with the onions, carrot, water, bay leaves, peppercorns, allspice berries, and cloves. Bake for 1 to 1½ hours, or until a thermometer inserted in the thickest part reads 167°F.

Remove the ham from the oven and allow it to cool completely. Then remove the ham from its broth. (Strain the broth and serve with rye bread for dunking.) You can refrigerate the ham overnight or immediately glaze and bake it.

When you're ready to glaze and bake the ham, preheat the oven to 450°F.

Whisk together the egg whites, brown sugar, and mustard in a small bowl. In another small bowl, whisk together the breadcrumbs and pepper.

Place the ham on a rimmed baking sheet. Trim off the skin and most of the fat. Brush it all over with the mustard glaze. With your hands, press the breadcrumbs onto the glazed ham.

Transfer the ham to a roasting pan and bake for about 10 minutes, until golden brown. Serve whole on the Christmas table, cold or slightly warm, and slice as needed.

Switzerland

Santa comes to Switzerland on December 6, known as Samichlaus Abend—Santa Night. Samichlaus wears a hooded red cape and long robe. His arrival marks the beginning of the Christmas season. He comes to town from a nearby forest rather than the North Pole, and children quickly gather around him as he arrives with his donkey, bearing gifts and treats.

But Samichlaus doesn't come alone. He travels with a mysterious sidekick called Schmutzli (Little Dirty One), who wears a dark and heavy hooded cape. His task is to "punish" naughty children by swatting them with a broom made of twigs. Samichlaus questions the children about their behavior in the past year and tries to get a commitment for improvement in the year ahead. Then *Lebkuchen,* chocolates, peanuts, and mandarins are delivered by the iconic pair, along with a *Grittibänz* (little bread man).

Throughout the season, towns are filled with bright colors, loud noises, clanging cowbells, glowing candles, and bellowing trumpets, creating a festive atmosphere and scaring away any evil Spirits that lurk during the dark days of winter.

Often, the Christmas tree is kept hidden away until Heiliger Abend (Holy Night, meaning Christmas Eve), and then is revealed after dinner. The children are delighted and surprised to see the tree adorned with Apples, bells, snowflakes, and sugar cookies. Many families still light their tree with real candles. The story of the Nativity is told, and the Austrian Christmas carol "Stille Nacht" (Silent Night) is sung. Then there is the hunting for hidden presents, followed by attendance at midnight Mass, where there is bell ringing and carol singing.

According to one folk tradition, on the very first Christmas when Jesus was born, animals were given the power to speak, a miracle that is repeated every year at midnight on Christmas Eve. Farm animals are given an extra portion of hay or grain on Heiliger Abend so that no one will accidentally overhear them speaking and thus invite a year of bad luck.[16]

The week between Christmas and New Year's Day is the time to visit neighbors and family, and delicious holiday pastries and cookies are on hand for the celebration. Popular sweets include *amaretti* (macaroon-type Almond-flavored cookies, originally from Italy), *änisbrötli* (Anise-flavored cookies with a stamped design), *basler läckerli* (hard spice cookies), *baumnuss guetzli* (Walnut cookies), *baumstriezel* (rolled dough that is wrapped around a stick and baked), Chestnuts (roasted over an open flame, soaked in syrup, or pureed and squeezed into strands of *vermicelles*), *christstollen* (pastry filled with fruit), *mohnstollen* (pastry filled with poppy seeds), *schaumküsse* (chocolate kisses), *grittibänz* (Christmas bread men), Lebkuchen (see the recipe on page 69), *pain d'epice* (honey and spice quick bread), *panettone* (see the recipe on page 84), and nougat.

Traditional holiday beverages are *glühwein* and *vin brulè*, made with red wine, mulling spices, and sometimes Raisins, served hot or warm; the first recorded use of this mulled wine was by the Romans in the second century.[17]

The traditional Christmas dinner features items such as *filet im teig* (pastry-wrapped pork fillet with sausage meat), *fondue chinoise* (hot pot), and *schinkli im teig* (pastry-wrapped hot ham) with potato salad.

✒ Swiss Baumnuss Guetzli (Walnut Cookies)

Makes about 40 cookies

For the Cookies
2 extra-large free-range organic egg whites
Pinch of sea salt
¾ cup organic sugar
²/₃ cup hazelnuts
1 cup walnuts
Organic flour, for dusting the work surface

For the Glaze
²/₃ cup organic confectioners' (powdered) sugar
1½ tablespoons organic cream
½ teaspoon pure almond extract
Pinch of sea salt
Whole walnut halves, for decorating

Make the Cookies

Combine the egg whites and salt in a medium metal bowl and beat until stiff.

Combine the sugar and nuts in a food processor or coffee grinder and pulse until the nuts are finely ground, with a texture almost like flour. Fold the sweetened nut mixture into the egg whites to form a sticky dough.

On a floured work surface, roll out the dough to about ¼-inch thickness.

Adapted from "Walnut Cookies (Baumnuss Guetzli) Recipe, Gourmetpedia (website), accessed January 28, 2021.

Use cookie cutters (a star shape is traditional) to cut out shapes, or cut them by hand. Place the cookies on a baking sheet lined with parchment paper.

Cover the cookies and allow them to rest for at least 4 hours and up to overnight.

Preheat the oven to 350°F.

Bake the cookies for about 10 minutes, until lightly golden. Let cool on a wire rack.

Make the Glaze

Combine the confectioners' sugar, cream, almond extract, and salt and stir until smooth. Spoon the glaze into a plastic ziplock bag and snip off one corner so you can squeeze out the icing. Top each cookie with icing, then place a whole walnut on top. Let dry.

Venezuela

The Venezuelan Christmas season begins on December 16 with an early-morning Mass (*misa de aguinaldo*), which is held again every morning until December 24. Each morning firecrackers are lit and bells ring to wake worshippers before dawn. Neighborhoods close the streets to cars until after Mass and then everyone enjoys *tostados* (toast) and coffee.

Homes are decorated with colored lights and an elaborate Nacimiento (Nativity scene) depicting mountains, hills, plains, and valleys. The focus of the Nacimiento is the *pesebre* (manger), featuring figures of Mary and Joseph and the animals that were in the stable with them. Adapting North American customs, some homes may erect artificial Christmas trees decorated with fake snow. Others paint a mural depicting a Christmas tree.[18]

Noche Buena ("Christmas Eve") is the Misa de Gallo (Mass of the Rooster). The name hearkens back to the time of the Romans who regarded cockcrow as the start of the day. After the Mass, families return home to enjoy a feast. At midnight firecrackers announce the coming of Christmas Day and the infant Jesus is placed in the pesebre. Baby Jesus is sung and prayed over and wine is drunk as gifts are opened.[19]

Young children receive presents twice, on December 25 and again on January 6 when the Three Kings are said to visit.

At Christmas time, revelers go from house to house singing *gaitas* (Christmas songs), accompanied by four string guitars and maracas. In some areas the Day of the Innocents is observed on December 28, a festival that commemorates the male infants killed by King Herod as he searched for the Messiah. There is music, dancing, costumes, and pranks.[20]

Venezuelan Christmas fare includes dishes such as turkey or chicken, *hallaca* (pork, beef, or chicken and vegetables wrapped in plantain leaves), *tamales* (cornmeal dough stuffed with meat, Onions, Garlic, and Chiles, wrapped in corn husks, and steamed), *pan de jamon* (bread filled with cooked ham and Raisins), and *dulce de lechoza* (a cold dessert made with green Papaya and brown sugar), salads, vegetables, and fruits.

🌶 Hallacas Caraqueñas (Caracas Tamales)

The filling for these traditional Venezuelan tamales is a meaty guiso, or stew, with achiote (annatto) seeds. Achiote is a favorite food coloring in Latin America; it has a strong flavor, so use sparingly. The wrappings are plantain leaves, which you can find in most major grocery stores and in Latin and Asian stores. Make sure the leaves are smoked; raw leaves will break when being folded.

Makes about 20 hallacas

For the Achiote Oil
1½ cups organic extra-virgin olive oil
4½ tablespoons achiote seeds

For the Filling
2½ pounds boneless organic beef chuck roast
2½ pounds skinless, boneless organic chicken breasts
2 teaspoons kosher salt, plus extra as desired
12 cups water
3 medium organic tomatoes, coarsely chopped
3 organic garlic cloves

Adapted from Claudia Martinez's "Hallacas," reproduced on the *Bon Appétit* website from its December 2020 issue, accessed February 5, 2021.

1 (6-ounce) can organic tomato paste

1 medium organic onion, chopped

1 large organic red bell pepper, seeds and ribs removed, coarsely chopped

1 large organic green bell pepper, seeds and ribs removed, coarsely chopped

1 bunch cilantro, coarsely chopped

1 bunch scallions, coarsely chopped

¼ cup packed organic light brown sugar

½ cup achiote oil

For the Dough

1 (1-kilogram) package precooked cornmeal (slightly more than 2 pounds)

1½ tablespoons kosher salt

8 cups water

1 cup achiote oil

For Assembly

3 (1-pound) packages banana or plantain leaves, fresh or frozen and thawed

¼ cup organic extra-virgin olive oil

1 cup water

½ cup drained capers

½ cup pitted green olives

½ cup organic raisins

Make the Achiote Oil

Combine the oil and achiote seeds in a small saucepan over medium-low heat. Cook until the oil turns deep orange, about 10 minutes. Strain into a heatproof jar and let cool.

Make the Filling

Combine the beef, chicken, salt, and 12 cups water in a large pot over medium-high heat. Bring to a boil, then reduce the heat to medium-low and let simmer until the meat is cooked through, about 30 minutes. Using a slotted spoon, transfer the beef and chicken to a cutting board and let it sit until cool enough to handle.

Pour 8 cups of the cooking liquid into a heatproof container and set aside. Discard the remaining liquid.

Cut the beef and chicken into $^1/_3$-inch cubes and place them back in the pot.

Combine the tomatoes, garlic, and tomato paste in a blender and blend until smooth. Scrape the puree into the pot with the meat.

Combine the onion, red and green bell peppers, cilantro, scallions, and ½ cup of the reserved cooking liquid in the blender. Blend until smooth and add to the pot.

Add the brown sugar and achiote oil to the pot. Pour in the remaining 7½ cups of reserved cooking liquid. Bring to a boil, then reduce heat to medium-low and simmer until the meat is tender and the liquid is slightly reduced, about 40 minutes.

Drain the meat in a colander, season lightly with salt, and let cool.

Make the Dough

Combine the cornmeal, salt, water, and achiote oil in a large bowl. Mix with your hands until the dough is smooth and spreadable and no large lumps remain, 5 to 7 minutes. Press a sheet of plastic wrap or parchment paper directly onto the surface of the dough. Let it rest for at least 30 minutes and up to 1 hour.

Assemble the Hallacas

Wash and pat the banana leaves dry. Use kitchen shears to carefully remove any center stems, avoiding breaking through the leaves. Then cut the leaves into 14-inch by 10-inch rectangles.

Mix the olive oil and water in a medium bowl that is big enough to dip your hands into. This will help keep the dough from sticking to your hands.

Working one at a time, place a banana leaf on a work surface so the veins in the leaves run horizontally. Dipping your hands in the oil mixture as you work, place ¾ cup dough in the center of a leaf and spread it out with your fingers into a $^1/_8$-inch-thick rectangle, leaving a 1-inch border near the vertical edges and a space on both horizontal edges.

Place ¾ cup of the filling in the center of dough. Top with five capers, two olives, and eight raisins.

Take the top and bottom edges of the leaf and them bring up toward each other, so the edges of the dough meet and enclose the filling; then pull them together toward the upper edge of the hallaca to seal it, and fold them over toward you, enclosing the filling in a leaf tube. Fold the two sides in toward the center to make a small package.

Place the package, fold side down, on another banana leaf and wrap it up again. Wrap once more in a third leaf to hold everything together, then tie the package closed with kitchen twine. (Make sure the package is compact, the leaves are not ripped, and hallaca is not leaking.)

Repeat with remaining dough, filling, and banana leaves.

Cook the Hallacas

Place as many hallacas as will fit into a large pot, pour in water to cover, and bring to a boil. Reduce the heat and simmer, turning the hallacas halfway through, until plumped and firm, about 35 minutes.

Repeat with the remaining hallacas.

Serve warm, or let them cool, then cover and store in the refrigerator for up to 1 week, or freeze for up to 3 months. To reheat, cook in a pot of simmering water (make sure the hallacas are submerged), partially covered, until warmed through, 10 to 15 minutes if chilled, or 25 to 30 minutes if frozen.

Wales

On the day of Y Nadolig (Christmas), there is a very early candlelight church service, known as *Plygain* (which means "daybreak"), between 4 a.m. and 6 a.m., when the Sun rises. The service is interspersed with carols, sometimes sung in three- or four-part harmony. Afterward, a day of feasting begins.

The pre-Christian ritual of the Mari Lwyd (Gray Mare) originates in Wales, and is being revived in many areas. (See page 30 for more on the Mari Lwyd.)

It is customary here to take down the Christmas greenery and remove the remnants of the Yule Log from the fireplace on Twelfth Night (January 5).[21]

Traditional Christmas fare can include smoked salmon, a turkey or goose roast, *cawl* (a stew made from ham, goose, lamb, or beef and Leeks), Potatoes and other root vegetables, mince pies, cheeses, savory biscuits, chutneys, Christmas cake, homemade toffee, and *pwdin Dolig* (Christmas pudding).

🍃 Welsh Cawl

Use a cheaper cut of meat on the bone for maximum flavor. You can also serve the meat separately to the vegetable soup.

Makes 6 servings

2¼ pounds organic middle neck or shoulder of Welsh
    lamb or beef, or a ham hock
1 organic onion, roughly chopped
6 medium organic potatoes, peeled and chopped
3 organic carrots, peeled and chopped
1 small organic rutabaga or 2 organic parsnips, peeled
    and chopped
2 organic leeks, washed and sliced
1 small bunch fresh parsley, roughly chopped
Organic vegetable stock, if needed
Sea salt and freshly ground black pepper, to taste

Place the meat in a large pot, cover with water, and bring to the boil, then simmer for 2 to 3 hours over low heat. Let cool, then transfer to the refrigerator to chill overnight. The following day, skim off any fat that has risen to the surface.

Cut the meat off the bone and return it to the stock. Add the potatoes, carrots, rutabaga or parsnips. Bring to a boil, then reduce the heat and simmer until the vegetables have softened.

Add vegetable stock, if needed. Season with salt and pepper. Add the sliced leeks. Cook until everything is warmed through. Just before serving, throw in the chopped parsley.

Adapted from Dudley Newbury's "How to Make Cawl," Visit Wales (website), accessed February 1, 2021.

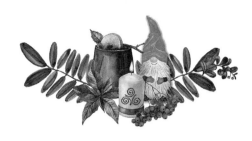

WASSAILING AND OTHER YULETIDE LIBATIONS

Wassail and wassail all over the town,
The cup it is white and the ale it is brown;
The cup it is made of the good old ashen tree,
And so is our beer of the best barley.
To you a wassail!
Aye, and joy come to our jolly wassail.

O maid, O maid, with your silver-headed pin,
Pray open the door and let us all in,
All for to fill our wassail-bowl and so away again.
To you a wassail!
Aye, and joy come to our jolly wassail.

O maid, O maid, with your glove and your mace,
Pray come unto this door and show your pretty face,
For we are truly weary of standing in this place.
To you a wassail!
Aye, and joy come to our jolly wassail.

O master and mistress, if you are so well pleased
Pray set all on your table your white bread and cheese,
And put forth your roast beef, your porrops and your pies.

To you a wassail!
Aye, and joy come to our jolly wassail.

O master and mistress, if we've done any harm,
Pray pull fast this door and let us pass along,
And give us hearty thanks for singing of our song.
To you a wassail!
Aye, and joy come to our jolly wassail.

"WASSAIL SONG," COLLECTED AND ARRANGED BY
CECIL J. SHARP IN *ONE HUNDRED ENGLISH*
FOLKSONGS (1916)

Wassailing is an English practice of going from house to house, singing carols and drinking to people's health. The word *wassail* comes from the Saxon *waes hael* (good health). The proper reply is *drinc heil* (drink well). To wassail is to drink to someone's health, especially from a decorated bowl. The drink itself is also called wassail.

According to legend, Vortigern, prince of the Silures, a pre-Roman Celtic tribe, fell in love with Rowena, the niece of Hengist, a Saxon king. She presented him with a bowl of spiced wine, saying, "Waes heal, Hlaford Cyning" (Be of health, Lord King). Vortigern married her, and his kingdom was eventually conceded to the Saxons—and the name for and practice of that kingdom-worthy wine came down to us through the ages.

The wassail bowl is a seasonal Yuletide object. The traditional wassail drink is "lamb's wool" (see the recipe on page 118), which is spiced ale with roasted apples.[1] The bowl is often decorated with ribbons and branches of Rosemary and is carried by girls, sometimes called "wassail wenches" or "vessel maids," who sing carols as they process around town. In Yorkshire, the bowl is called the "vessel cup" and is decorated with Holly and evergreens. Wassailers go from door to door offering a drink and expecting a tip.

Inside the home, a wassail bowl of hot spiced ale with toast, apples, or Christmas cake floating in it is served. Guests stir the hot ale with a silver spoon while walking around the brew Sunwise (clockwise).

Wassailing can begin as early as November, and the usual pattern is for two "vessel maids" to carry a box decorated with evergreens and covered with a white cloth from house to house. Arriving at the door, the girls sing and then ask for a coin to reveal what lies under the cloth. One description of the contents is two dolls (a larger one dressed in red and a smaller doll), some paper flowers, Holly and Mistletoe, a purse with a hole in it, an Apple, an Orange, and sweets. The box is lined with Ivy and Moss, and the dolls represent the Virgin and Child.[2]

Wassailing the Trees

Wassail the trees that they may bear
You many a plum and many a pear;
For more or less fruits they will bring,
as you do give them wassailing.

On Christmas Eve, Devonshire farm families go to the orchard with a large jug of cider and drink a toast to the best-bearing Apple trees, firing guns and making a loud racket. The noise is meant to scare off malevolent Spirits and to encourage (or frighten!) the trees into producing a good crop of Apples in the coming season.

In Somersetshire, each person in the company takes a cupful of cider, drinks part of the contents, and throws the rest at the tree.[3]

Pieces of toast soaked in cider are hung in the branches of the largest Apple tree for the robins, who represent the good Spirits of the tree.

Here's to thee, old apple tree, that blooms well,
bears well.
Hats full, caps full, three-bushel bags full, And all
under one tree.
Hurrah. Hurrah![4]

In some areas, fruit trees are beaten with sticks and entreated to be fruitful. (Oddly, I was once assured by a native Californian man that the same treatment is essential if you want a healthy avocado crop!)

In Cornwall, a song is sung while holding a jug of ale in one hand and a stick in the other:

Huzza, huzza in our good town
The bread shall be white, and the liquor be brown,
So here my old fellow I drink to thee
And the very health of each other tree.
Well may ye blow, well may ye bear
Blossom and fruit, both apple and pear.
So that every bough and every twig
May bend with a burden both fair and big
May ye ever bear us and yield us fruit such a store
That the bags and chambers and house run o'er.

In southern Hampshire, the wassailers are more threatening:

Apple tree,
Apple tree,
Bear good fruit,
Or down with your top
And up with your root!

Other countries follow similar customs. In Romania, for example, a farmer carries an ax, accompanied by his wife with her hands covered in dough. The farmer visits each barren tree and threatens to cut it down. The wife responds, saying; "Oh, I am sure this tree will be as full of fruit in the spring as my fingers are with dough today."

Wassailing the Animals

In the West Country, farmers might wassail the oxen on Twelfth Night. Men and women go to the barn, sip from the wassail bowl, take a cake from a basket ornamented with greenery, and impale it on an ox's horns. If the ox remains quiet, that signals very good luck.

In Sussex and Hertfordshire, celebrants wassail the beehives.[5]

🌿 Lamb's Wool (Hot Mulled Beer or Ale with Apples)

Long ago, wassail was made with cream and egg whites, which were whipped, leading to frothing that looks like the white wool of a lamb—and that is thought to be the origin of the peculiar "lamb's wool" name for this traditional Yuletide beverage.[6]

Makes 6–8 servings

> 3 organic apples, peeled, cored, and finely chopped
> 3 tablespoons organic butter
> 3 (12-ounce) bottles dark beer
> ½ cup firmly packed organic brown sugar
> 1 teaspoon ground cinnamon
> 1 teaspoon ground ginger
> ½ teaspoon ground nutmeg

Preheat the oven to 350°F.

Place the apples and butter in a baking dish. Bake for 30 minutes.

Combine the baked apples in a large saucepan with the beer, brown sugar, and spices. Heat until just hot and serve.

Adapted from Bergy's "Lamb's Wool (Hot Mulled Beer with Apples)," Food.com (website), accessed May 10, 2021.

More Yuletide Libations

Here is a selection of decadent celebratory drinks from other cultures that can be incorporated into your own festive Yuletide gathering.

🌿 Chilean Aguardiente Coffee Eggnog: Cola de Mono para Navidad (Monkey Tail for Christmas)

Kitchen Witches and Hearth Druids take note: Coffee has many magical aspects. It is grounding (pun intended), helps you get to work and finish projects, and can help remove negativity. As a stimulant, it enhances and speeds the action of potions, charms, and spells and is used to speedily break curses and remove obstacles.

Adapted from Maricel Presilla's "Chilean Aguardiente Coffee Eggnog: Cola de Mono para Navidad," Food Network (website), accessed May 13, 2021.

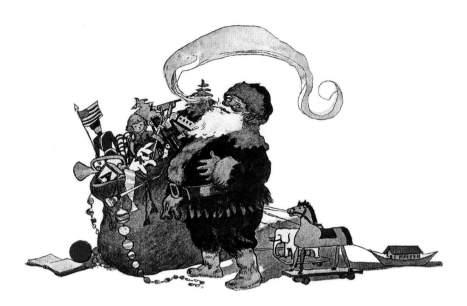

Plate 1. American Santa. In the nineteenth century, Santa Claus, whose
name and attributes descend directly from those of Saint Nicholas, became
a fabled gift bringer in the lore of the United States.
By Jessie Wilcox Smith (1863–1935). Original from The New York Public Library.

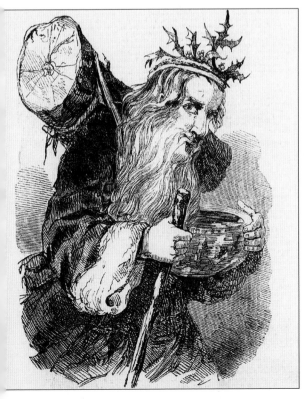

Plate 2. Father Christmas with
a Yule Log on his back and a
wassail bowl in his hands.
*By Alfred Crowquill, 1848, The
Illustrated London News.*

Plate 3. Jultomte. The Swedish Jultomte, Norwegian Julenisse, Danish Julemand, and Finnish Joulupukki (each name translates roughly to "Christmas Elf") is a Spirit, Gnome, or Pixie-like character that helps with chores in the house and on the farm. At Christmas time, they bring gifts for their households. *Christmas card by Jenny Nyström.*

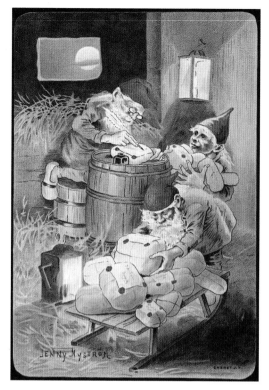

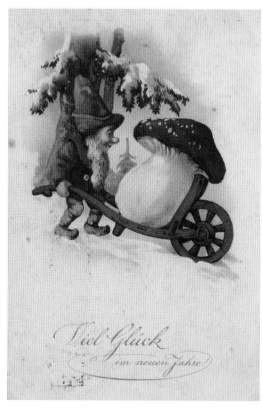

Plate 4. Figures of red-capped Nisser (house Elves) and red-and-white-spotted Amanita mushrooms are featured in Scandinavian Christmas decorations. Some say Santa is an incarnation of a shamanic mushroom Spirit, seen by Siberian shamans when they partake of *Amanita muscaria.* This mushroom may be the reason why Santa is dressed in red and white. *Image from the 1900s.*

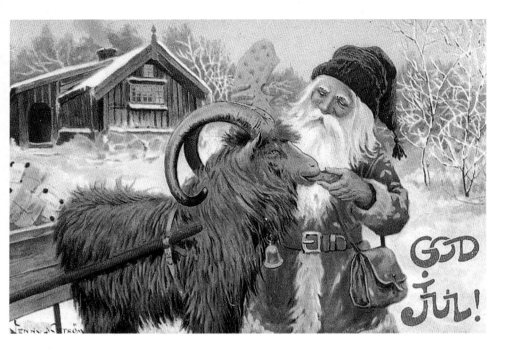

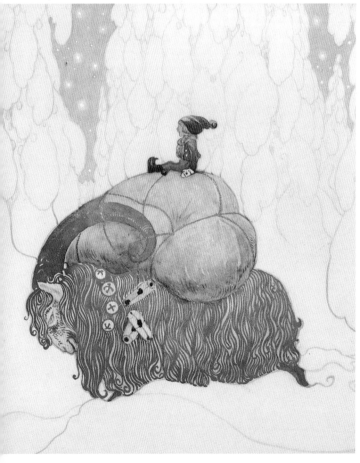

Plates 5 and 6. In some parts of Sweden, the Julbukk (Yule buck or Christmas goat) brings gifts, pulling a Jultomte with a red cap and long white beard. This story echoes the mythology of ancient Pagan Scandinavia in which two goats pulled the God Thor across the sky, adding a mystical dimension to the Christmas Goat. *Postcard by Jenny Nyström. Julbocken by John Bauer, 1912.*

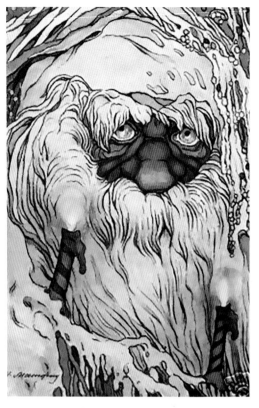

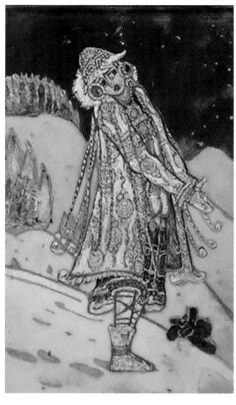

Plates 7 (top left) and 8 (top right). The Russian New Year's is when Ded Moroz (Grandfather Frost) brings presents to children. He has a long white beard and carries a big magic staff as a symbol of his power. He is always accompanied by his granddaughter Snegurochka (Snow Maiden). On New Year's Eve, children hold hands, make a circle around the Christmas tree, and call for Snegurochka or Ded Moroz. *Ded Moroz postcard by Matorin Nikolay Vasilyevich. Snegurochka, Nicholas Roerich, 1912.*

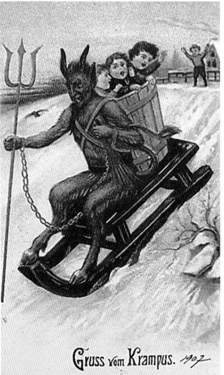

Gruss vom Krampus. 1907

Plate 9. In lower Austria, Saint Nicholas is accompanied by Krampus, a horned Demon carrying a whip. He has a basket on his back in which to capture bad children. *190*

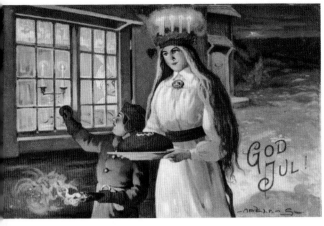

Plate 10. Lucia, the light bearer, is celebrated in Scandinavia, Italy, Slovenia, and Croatia. In Scandinavia on December 13, Saint Lucia's Day, young girls in white dresses with crowns of lights (or candles) on their heads carry candles, cookies, and Saffron buns in procession as shown here.
Christmas card by Adèle Söderberg, circa 1916.

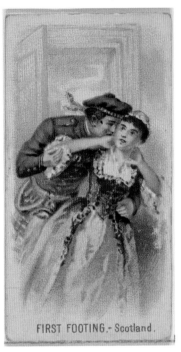

FIRST FOOTING.- Scotland.

Plate 11. In Scotland, Wales, and other parts of Europe, the first person to cross the threshold of the house after the stroke of midnight on Christmas Eve or on New Year's Eve—The First Footing—determines the fortunes of the family in the year to come. The most desirable visitor is a dark, handsome, single male.
First Footing, Scotland, from the Holidays series (N80) for Duke brand cigarettes MET DPB883117, 1890.

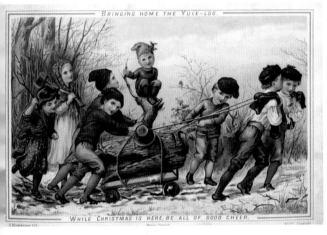

Plate 12. The tradition of the Yule log—continuously burning a large piece of wood in the hearth (which other than key holes is the only vulnerable opening of the home where mischievous Spirits might enter) throughout the Winter Solstice and Christmas season—was first known in the Italian Alps, Balkans, Scandinavia, France, and Iberia. By saving a piece of the log all year, the family carries the protection through to the next Yuletide.
Victorian Christmas card from Nova Scotia archives.

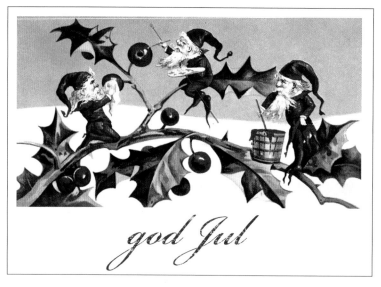

Plate 13. Elves painting berries on holly leaves. *From The Miriam and Ira D. Wallach Division Of Art, Prints and Photographs: Picture Collection published by L. Prang & Co. Original From The New York Public Library.*

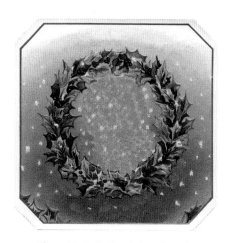

Plate 14. In Ireland the door is decorated with a Holly wreath. Fairy lights, Christmas trees, and other decorations are put up on December 8, the day of the Feast of the Immaculate Conception, and come down on "Little Christmas," or January 6. *Victoria Christmas card.*

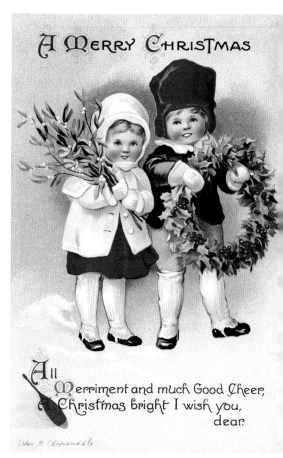

Plate 15. Children carrying Mistletoe and a Holly wreath. *By Ellen Clapsaddle.*

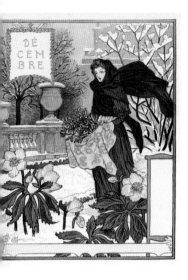

Plate 16. A woman gathering Mistletoe.
By Eugène Grasset, December, 1896.

Plate 17. The practice of setting up Christmas trees in the home appears to have originated in the early 1600s, perhaps in Strasburg, Germany. *Christmas Market in Nürnberg, Germany. Litography from the 19th century. Germanisches Nationalmuseum, Nürnberg, Germany.*

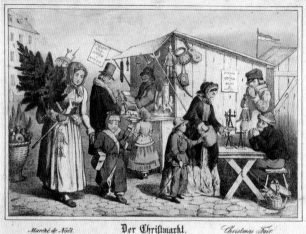

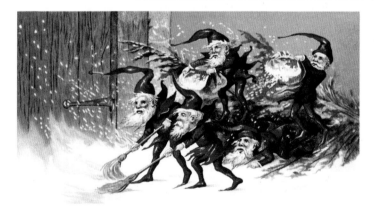

Plate 18. Elves sweeping snow with a Christmas tree in the background. *From The Miriam and Ira D. Wallach Division Of Art, Prints and Photographs: Picture Collection* published *by L. Prang & Co. Original From The New York Public Library.*

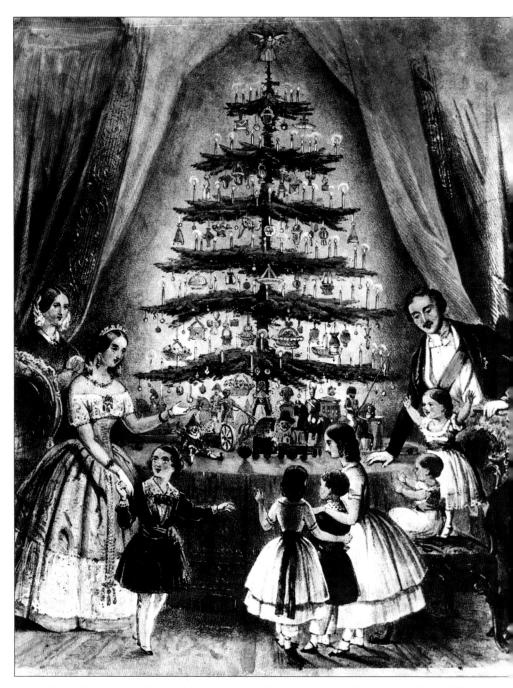

Plate 19. An 1848 illustration of Queen Victoria, Prince Albert, and their children admiring a Christmas tree. Many variations of this image circulated during this time and the trees became the rage with British families. Prince Albert, who loved everything about a traditional German Christmas, made a point of sending Christmas trees to schools and army barracks.
Image from 1848, photograph by Hulton Archive, Getty Images.

In some traditions, it is poured out as an offering to the Spirits and the ancestors. Think of these attributes as you add the instant coffee to this beverage.

Pisco is a type of brandy, about 38 to 48 proof. If you can't find it, look for a substitute with about the same alcohol content. White rum, a white brandy like grappa, or even a white tequila would work, though the taste won't be exactly the same.

This drink is best made the day before you intend to serve it.

Makes 12 servings

> 2 quarts organic whole milk
> ⅓ cup organic sugar
> 5 whole cloves
> 2 sticks cinnamon
> ½ vanilla bean, split and scraped
> ½ rind from an organic lemon
> ½ rind from an organic orange
> 1 tablespoon (or more if desired) organic instant coffee
>   dissolved in a little warm organic milk
> ½ bottle Chilean pisco

Combine the milk, sugar, cloves, cinnamon, vanilla, and lemon and orange peels in a pot over medium-high heat. Bring to a soft boil. As soon as the mixture boils, add the instant coffee mixture. Stir, cover, and remove from the heat. Let steep until cooled.

Strain into a bowl, then slowly stir in the pisco. Pour into a glass container and refrigerate.

🍂 Turkish Salep

Genuine salep flour is made from the ground tubers of wild orchids (Orchis mascula or Orchis militaris) that are found in southern Turkey and the Black Sea area. The plants are becoming endangered, so genuine salep flour is extremely hard to find outside Turkey, though salep-flavored sachets and powders can be had in North America. Genuine salep has health benefits, such as easing digestive

---

Adapted from Ozlem Warren's "Comforting Sahlep Drink with Cinnamon and Pistachio Nuts," *Ozlem's Turkish Table* (blog), March 5, 2015.

problems, helping with gum disease, and increasing resistance to coughs and colds. The drink made from it is traditionally served with ground cinnamon and ground pistachio nuts sprinkled on top.

Orchids are herbs of Venus. Kitchen Witches and Hearth Druids may be interested to know that fresh orchid roots promote true love, while the withered ones will check misguided passions.

Makes 2 servings

> 2 cups organic whole milk
>
> 1 tablespoon salep powder (or salep-flavored sachet)
>
> Organic sugar, to taste
>
> Ground cinnamon, for topping
>
> Ground pistachio nuts, for topping

Combine the milk, salep powder, and sugar in a nonaluminum pan and bring to a boil. Stir until the mix begins to thicken, 2 to 3 minutes. Remove from the heat and pour into cups. Serve hot, sprinkled with cinnamon and ground pistachios.

🍃 Nigerian Chapman Cocktail

A popular Nigerian drink. Make and serve immediately so as not to melt the ice and lose the fizz of the sodas. If serving to children, omit the bitters.

For Kitchen Witches and Hearth Druids, this citrusy beverage carries the bright energies of the Sun; cleansing, strength, joy, purification, happiness, and abundance are its gifts. The cucumber adds healing, fertility, beauty, and youthfulness to the brew.

Makes 4 servings

> 1$^1/_3$ cups chilled Fanta
>
> 1$^1/_3$ cups chilled Sprite
>
> 4–5 tablespoons black currant or Grenadine syrup
>
> ¼ teaspoon Angostura, Peychaud's, or orange bitters
>
> 1 organic lemon, sliced
>
> 1 organic orange, sliced
>
> 1 organic cucumber, sliced

Adapted from Lilian's "Nigerian Chapman: How to Make Chapman (Nigerian Special Cocktail)," Nigerian Food TV (website), accessed May 13, 2021.

Fill a large bowl with ice. Pour in the Fanta and Sprite, followed by the black currant or Grenadine syrup. Add the bitters and mix well. Fold in the lemon, orange, and cucumber slices.

Serve in tall cocktail glasses or large snifters, with slices of fruit and cucumber in each glass.

🍂 Korean Sujeonggwa: Dessert Punch with Persimmon, Cinnamon, and Ginger

Kitchen Witches and Hearth Druids take note: Persimmon is an herb of abundance (think of all the fruits), protection, longevity, love, healing, and luck. Cinnamon is an herb of purification that enhances psychic awareness, ignites passions, and ensures long-lasting love. Ginger increases personal power, kindles your sex life, and brings luck and healing.

Makes 4 or 5 servings

    ½ cup sliced organic ginger

    5 cinnamon sticks

    7½–8 cups water

    1 cup organic sugar or ½ cup raw, local honey

    4 or 5 dried organic persimmons

    Pine nuts, for topping

Combine the ginger, cinnamon, and water in a large nonaluminum pot over high heat. Cover, bring to a boil, and let boil for 20 minutes. Then lower the heat to medium and boil gently for another 25 minutes. (If it boils over, take off the lid for a moment.)

Stir in the sugar or honey, then remove from the heat and let cool.

Strain out the cinnamon sticks and sliced ginger. (Save them to add to black tea later!) Pour the strained liquid into a glass jar.

Remove the stems from the dried persimmons and wash the fruits thoroughly. Add them to the liquid in the jar. Put on a lid and chill in the refrigerator for at least 12 hours and up to 1 week.

Serve cold, over ice. Each serving should have one persimmon in it and a few pine nuts sprinkled on top.

Adapted from Maangchi's "Dessert Punch with Persimmon, Cinnamon, and Ginger," Maangchi (website), April 20, 2008.

🍃 Jamaican Sorrel: A Ruby-Red Christmas Drink

A cousin to the traditional African-American "red drink" (hibiscus tea), which itself derived from the bissap of African nations, sorrel is sometimes called agua de Jamaica in Latin American countries. It's said to have become a Christmas tradition in Jamaica because December is when the roselle hibiscus (Hibiscus sabdariffa) flowers.

Kitchen Witches and Hearth Druids will appreciate that hibiscus flowers are often used to make effective love potions. Deep red hibiscus stimulates both sexuality and passion.

Makes about 1½ quarts once diluted

> 2 cups whole, dried sorrel (dried hibiscus flowers)
> 2 inches fresh organic ginger, sliced thin for milder flavor, grated or mashed for stronger flavor
> Peel of 1 organic orange
> 2 cinnamon sticks
> 1 cup organic brown sugar, or to taste
> 6 cups water
> Rum, water, and ice, for serving

Combine the sorrel, ginger, orange peel, cinnamon, sugar, and water in a nonaluminum pot, cover, and bring to a gentle simmer. Let simmer for 30 minutes, then remove from the heat and let cool. Refrigerate at least overnight or for up to 3 days.

Strain the red liquid, and store in the refrigerator.

Serve over ice, diluted with water and mixed with rum as desired.

Adapted from Sasha Martin's "Jamaican Sorrel Drink," Global Table Adventure (website), accessed May 13, 2021.

🍃 Magical Yuletide Brandy Cocktail

Kitchen Witches and Hearth Druids will discern the cinnamon for vitality, allspice for healing, orange for joy, and lemon for purification. This empowering potion will enchant any Winter Solstice observance.

Adapted from Julia Halina Hadas's "Witchcraft Cocktails: Pomander and Brandy," *Witchology Magazine* no. 1, December 2020.

To make your own simple syrup, combine equal parts of sugar and water and simmer until the sugar is completely dissolved. The syrup will keep for up to 1 month when refrigerated in a closed container.

Makes 1 serving

> 2 tablespoons brandy
>
> 1 tablespoon orange liqueur, such as Cointreau or Orange Curaçao
>
> 1 tablespoon organic lemon juice
>
> 1 tablespoon organic orange juice
>
> 1 tablespoon allspice dram (see recipe below)
>
> 1 teaspoon simple syrup
>
> A pinch of ground cinnamon
>
> Curl of fresh organic orange peel, for garnish

Combine the brandy, orange liqueur, lemon and orange juices, allspice dram, simple syrup, and a pinch of cinnamon in a cocktail shaker (or a glass jar with a tight lid), along with some crushed ice. Visualize the returning sunlight and your own strengthening power and joy as you shake. Strain into a glass and garnish with a curl of orange peel.

Allspice Dram

This simple liqueur flavored with allspice berries is sometimes also known as pimento dram.

> $1/8$ cup whole allspice berries
>
> 1 cup light or dark rum
>
> 1 cinnamon stick
>
> $1\frac{1}{2}$ cups water
>
> $2/3$ cup organic brown sugar

Roughly crush the allspice berries with a mortar and pestle or coffee grinder, place in a glass jar, pour in the rum, shake, and let sit for 24 hours.

Snap the cinnamon stick into pieces and drop them into the jar. Let sit for 2 more days.

Strain the infused rum through cheesecloth or a coffee filter. Bring the water and sugar to a boil in a small saucepan. Boil for 5 minutes, cool, then mix into the rum. Pour into a bottle and let rest for 2 days before using.

🍃 Decadent Chocolate and Coffee Liqueur

The ancient Mayans called chocolate the "food of the Gods," and the Mayans and Aztecs used chocolate in ceremonies to become closer to the divine and to enhance a sense of connection and inspiration within the community. It was known to bring love, joy, and peace of mind, to enhance personal energy and creativity, and to enable those who consumed it to discover their true passion in life.

Whisk this liqueur with heavy cream and whiskey, mix it with chocolate syrup and pour it warm over vanilla ice cream, or add it to eggnog for a surprising twist. Make this in late summer or early fall to have it ready by Winter Solstice.

> 3 cups roasted organic coffee beans
> Whiskey
> Piece of honeycomb or 3 tablespoons raw, local honey
> 2 cinnamon sticks
> 1 teaspoon ground cloves

Place the beans under a cloth and crack them with a hammer, or grind them coarsely in a coffee grinder. Put the cracked beans into a glass jar and add enough whiskey to cover them. Drop in the honeycomb or honey, along with the cinnamon and cloves.

Let steep for at least 2 months in a cool, dark place. Shake the jar every few weeks to redistribute the ingredients.

Strain the liqueur and store in a tightly capped bottle or jar.

🍃 Hot Toddy with Herbs

Hot toddies are thought to have originated in Scotland. As Ross Dennis, of Dewar's Aberfeldy Distillery in Scotland, told an interviewer in 2016, "The first mention of what we now think of as a hot toddy comes about in the 1780s. We think the name hot toddy comes from the Todian Well, an ancient water source in Edinburgh."[7]

This tasty cold and flu remedy can be effective at the first sign of illness and will help you relax as you prepare for sleep. The original Scottish recipe is just whiskey, honey, and water, served in a crystal glass and stirred with a silver spoon.

Adapted from "5 Herbal Holiday Recipes," Traditional Medicinals (website), accessed May 14, 2021.

A cinnamon stick, a slice of ginger or lemon, or a few whole cloves are sometimes added.

In this herbal version, the slippery elm is soothing to a sore throat, while the licorice helps with a cough.

Makes 1 serving

> 1 cup water
> 1 tablespoon raw, local honey (heather honey would be ideal!)
> 1 bag slippery elm tea
> 1 bag licorice tea
> 9 teaspoons good single-malt whiskey
> ¼ cup organic lemon juice (or one large wedge of lemon,
>   squeezed into the cup)

Bring the water to the boil. Place the honey in a large mug, along with the tea bags. Pour in the water, cover the mug with a saucer, and let steep for 10 minutes.

Uncover, remove the tea bags, and add the whiskey and lemon. Stir well.

Set a silver spoon in a fine crystal glass.* Pour in the hot drink, stir, and sip slowly.

---

*The silver spoon prevents the glass from cracking.

🌿 Ginger and Honey Hot Toddy

Ginger root has antibacterial properties, the honey soothes a cough, and the lemon provides vitamin C. This warming brew is ideal before bed or before a hot bath so you can "sweat out" an illness.

Makes 1 serving.

> 2 inches fresh organic ginger, cut into coins
> 1 cup water
> A quarter of an organic lemon (or ¼ cup organic lemon juice)
> 1 tablespoon raw, local honey (heather honey would be ideal!)
> 3 tablespoons good single-malt whiskey

Combine the ginger slices and water in a nonaluminum pot with a tight lid. Simmer for 20 minutes.

Set a silver spoon into a fine crystal glass. Strain the hot liquid into the glass. Add the honey and lemon and stir well. Add the whiskey and sip slowly.

Note: Ginger has a very sturdy volatile oil, so the same slices of root can be used twice to make tea.

Herb-Infused Winter Gin

This one will make you feel you are drinking a forest. Gin gets its distinctive flavor from juniper berries; this version builds upon it with conifer and other winter flavors. Make this recipe at least a week before Solstice and serve it to your Coven or Grove.

For the conifer, take care not to use yew (it's poisonous) or commercially grown Christmas trees (they're sprayed with pesticides).

Makes 16 servings

> 2 tablespoons fresh or dried juniper berries
>
> 3 cups vodka or other neutral tasting spirit
>
> 3-inch sprig of fresh white fir, pine, spruce, blue spruce, or another edible conifer
>
> 2 teaspoons coriander seeds or aniseeds
>
> 1 teaspoon dried or fresh grated organic orange peel
>
> 1 whole allspice berry
>
> 1 cinnamon stick
>
> 1 fresh or dried sage leaf
>
> ½ dried California bay leaf or 1 dried Turkish bay leaf

Put the juniper berries in a quart jar and pour the vodka over them. Cap tightly and let infuse for at least 12 hours.

Add the rest of the herbs and spices, cap, and let infuse for 36 hours.

Strain the infused gin, using a fine-mesh sieve or cheesecloth. Store in a bottle or jar in a cool and dark place for up to 1 year.

Serve well iced, with a sprig of Yuletide greenery in each glass.

Adapted from Colleen Codekas's "Homemade Infused Gin: Foraged Botanical Winter Spirits," *Grow Forage Cook Ferment* (blog), November 17, 2020.

🍂 Rosy Red Pomegranate Solstice Martini

Pomegranates are sacred to the Goddess Persephone, who is the daughter of Demeter, the Goddess of fertility and the harvest, and of Zeus. Most people are familiar with her story: Hades abducted Persephone and carried her off to the Underworld. She was understandably distraught and suffering, but Hades slyly fed her a few pomegranate seeds, knowing that anyone who ate food in the Underworld was compelled to return there. So, when Zeus finally interceded, forcing Hades to return Persephone to her mother Demeter, he decreed that Persephone could spend only half the year with her mother on Olympus, and the other half of the year she would spend with Hades in the Underworld. Now, when Persephone is gone from her, Demeter mourns, and the Earth becomes cold and dark. When she returns to her mother, the plants and flowers flourish and the world rejoices.[8]

A word to the wise: As everyone knows (or should know), if you consume any food or drink while visiting the Underworld or the Fairy realm, you will be doomed to return or to stay there. So don't do it!

Pomegranate is a female plant—the fruit resembles ovaries filled with eggs (the seeds), and the juice looks like blood. Pomegranate will help enhance female, nurturing qualities in both men and women. Drink pomegranate juice to put yourself in resonance with Goddesses.

Rosemary is an herb of purification. It is masculine in nature and ruled by the Sun, making it a perfect herb for invoking the Sun at the Winter Solstice.

Drink a pomegranate libation at Solstice in honor of Persephone, soon to be liberated to walk in the warm spring sunlight once more.

Makes 1 large serving or 2 smaller ones

For the Rosemary Honey Syrup
½ cup raw, local honey
½ cup water
1 or 2 sprigs very fresh and fragrant rosemary

For the Martini
3 tablespoons gin (or other spirit of choice, such as
  tequila, rum, or vodka)

Adapted from Colleen Codekas's "Pomegranate Martini with Rosemary Honey Syrup," *Grow Forage Cook Ferment* (blog), December 23, 2019.

  1 tablespoon citrus liqueur. such as Orange Curaçao or
  Cointreau
  $\frac{1}{8}$ cup rosemary honey syrup
  1 tablespoon freshly squeezed organic lime juice
  4 tablespoons organic pomegranate juice
  1 fresh rosemary sprig, for garnish

Make the Rosemary Honey Syrup

Combine the honey, water, and rosemary sprigs in a pot and bring to a simmer over medium heat. Stir well, then remove from the heat. Steep, covered, until the liquid cools to room temperature. Strain the liquid through a sieve, pour into a jar with a tight lid, and store in the refrigerator for up to 2 weeks.

Make the Martini

Combine the gin, citrus liqueur, syrup, lime juice, and pomegranate juice in a cocktail shaker (or a glass jar with a tight lid). Add crushed ice and shake well. Strain into a martini glass. Garnish with a sprig of fresh rosemary.

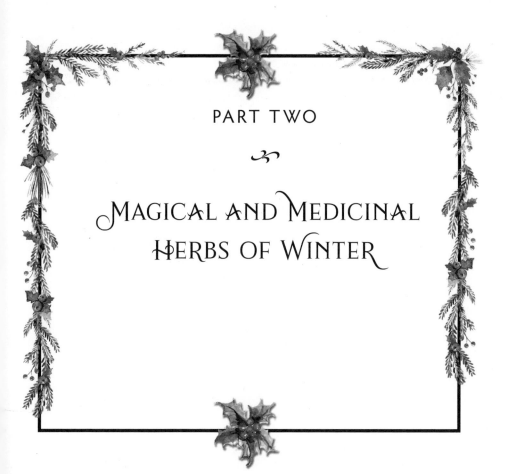

PART TWO

❧

MAGICAL AND MEDICINAL
HERBS OF WINTER

The plants profiled in this chapter all have a special connection with Yuletide and Christmas, and all are valuable winter medicines. Roots, barks, berries, leaves, flowers, nuts, and seeds have many dimensions and spectrums of influence. As you work with each one, whether in cooking, ritual, or medicine, think also of the spiritual qualities and magic the plant embodies.

Allspice
(Pimenta dioica)

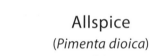

Allspice, native to the West Indies and Central America, came to the attention of the wider world after early European explorers encountered it. The British called the berries "allspice" because of their flavor, which is reminiscent of a combination of Clove, Pepper, Cinnamon, and Nutmeg. Sometimes the plant is called Jamaican Pepper. There is nothing like the scent of spiced cookies, cakes, and brews wafting through the home to put you in the mood for the Yuletide season.

Medicinal Properties

Allspice leaves and berries are antibacterial, hypotensive (lowering blood pressure), antineuralgic (relieving nerve pain), and analgesic (relieving pain). They also are strong antioxidants. They have potent effects against prostate and breast cancers and can help relieve menopausal discomforts.

In Jamaica, Allspice is commonly added to teas for colds, menstrual cramps, and indigestion. The berries are used for dyspepsia and diabetes in Costa Rica. They are crushed and applied as a poultice to bruises, sore joints, and muscle aches in Guatemala; and they're mixed with other herbs for indigestion in Cuba.

Ayurvedic doctors use the berries to relieve chest congestion and toothache.

Herbalists add Allspice essential oil to massage oils and baths because it is known to promote circulation and to relieve pain from muscle cramps, strains, and rheumatism. They also use Allspice to relieve headache, stress, depression, and fatigue.[1]

To make a tea: Steep ½ teaspoon of ground Allspice per cup of freshly boiled water, covered, for 10 minutes, then strain. Take ¼ cup four times a day.

To make a poultice: Mix ground Allspice with just enough water to make a thick paste. Spread the paste on a clean cloth and apply for 20 minutes.

For a massage oil or liniment: Mix 2 or 3 drops of Allspice essential oil with 3 tablespoons of a carrier oil, such as Grapeseed, Coconut, or Olive oil, and massage it into the painful area. Wash hands thoroughly afterward. Take care to not get the oil into your eyes or mucous membranes. Do *not* ingest the essential oil.[2]

> **CAUTION: Allspice can irritate the skin of sensitive persons, and it can slow blood clotting. Stop using it at least 2 weeks before a scheduled surgery. Pregnant and breastfeeding women can safely use Allspice as a culinary spice but should probably avoid medicinal amounts. Overuse could lead to an upset stomach.[3]**

Magical Uses
An herb of Mars, Allspice is used as whole berries or ground. Add it to healing incenses and to Spirit bags and charms. It attracts abundance, money, luck, and healing.

Allspice at Yuletide
Add the ground berries to your Winter Solstice incense. Use the spice in cookies and other seasonal dishes to bring luck in the new Sun cycle.

🜄 Spiced Dutch Baby Pancakes for a Winter Breakfast

Makes 1 pancake (enough for at least 2 servings)

3 free-range organic eggs

¾ cup organic milk (or unsweetened almond or oat milk)

½ cup unbleached organic flour (wheat or gluten-free)

Pinch of sea salt

1 teaspoon pure vanilla extract

1 teaspoon ground cinnamon

¼ teaspoon ground allspice

¼ teaspoon ground nutmeg

⅛ teaspoon ground cardamom

1 tablespoon organic unsalted butter

For Serving

Maple syrup

Dried cranberries

Pecans

Organic confectioners' (powdered) sugar

Place an oven-safe 10-inch skillet (such as a cast-iron pan) into the oven, and preheat the oven to 475°F.

Beat the eggs and milk until frothy, using an electric mixer or a wire whisk. Slowly whisk in the flour, salt, vanilla, and spices and beat for a minute or so.

When the oven is very hot, remove the skillet and reduce the oven heat to 425°F.

Place the butter in the hot skillet and swirl it around until the butter is melted and the skillet is coated. Pour the batter into the skillet and immediately return it to the oven. Bake the pancake for about 15 minutes, until golden and puffy.

Serve with maple syrup, dried cranberries, a sprinkling of pecans, and a dusting of confectioners' sugar.

Adapted from "Winter Spiced Dutch Baby Pancake with Pecan Maple Syrup," a Kitchenaid recipe posted on Yummly (website), accessed May 19, 2021.

Almond
(*Prunus dulcis*)

..................✼....................

*They set up for themselves pillars and Asherim on every
high hill and under every green tree.*

2 KINGS 17:10

The ancient Semites were polytheistic worshippers of nature who saw
their highest Goddess in the form of a tree: the flowering Almond.
Almond trees give of themselves in many ways, providing nourishment
in their fruits and heralds of spring in their delicate blossoms. In their
beauty, the ancients saw the qualities of the Goddess Asherah, blessing
Her people with sustenance and grace.

At that time, Yahweh was one of several male deities, including Baal, El,
and Hadad. The Goddess was known as Asherah, Anash, Qedesh, or Elah,
the feminine aspect of El. A pillar or pole, as a representation of Asherah/
Elah, would be set up on a high place, an artificial platform or altar, or on a
hill, if at all possible, in desert areas where trees would not grow. The pillar
was erected with a bust or face of the Goddess placed on top.

So important was the flowering Almond tree in the minds of the
people that even after the monotheistic, patriarchal Yahwistic religion
took over, the memory of Asherah was kept holy. Ancient biblical scrip-
ture specified that the menorah, the candelabrum of the time of the
Winter Solstice and the darkest Moon of the year, must look like a flowering Almond tree with buds on its branches. A chief cult of Yahweh
lit its menorah on all-important occasions, and as it was forbidden to
depict or even to name Yahweh in any physical form, so it was forbidden to depict the menorah, symbol of the deity in female aspect. Thus,
the earliest images come to us from Roman times, when the conquering
Latins carved a menorah onto a triumphal arch.[4]

In modern times, the menorah is lit during the dark of the Moon
in the darkest season of winter. As the Moon waxes, another candle is
lit each evening, until on the final night all eight branches are ignited,
symbolically bringing back the light.

Marzipan, a classic Christmas sweet made from ground Almonds, egg white, and sugar, may derive from the Arabic *mawthaban* and was most likely brought to medieval Europe by returning Crusaders. In the Tudor era, when it was known as marchpane, it was shaped into fruits, flowers, vegetables, animals, and other forms as candy and for Christmas decorations.

Medicinal Properties

Medicinally, Almonds can help reduce heart disease risk by lowering total and LDL cholesterol levels. They are anti-inflammatory and anti-oxidant and rich in unsaturated fat. In clinical trials they have been shown to promote healthy blood vessels and to reduce insulin resistance.[5] Almonds are very beneficial to the brain, enhancing memory and reducing headaches, cognitive decline, and brain fog.

Eating more nuts in general, including Almonds, can reduce the risk of cardiovascular disease, cancer, and deaths from other causes overall.[6]

CAUTION: Diabetics should watch for signs of low blood sugar and monitor their blood sugar carefully if eating Almonds in volume. Eating large amounts of Almonds could worsen pain and diarrhea in people with irritable bowel syndrome (IBS). Avoid drinking large amounts of Almond milk if your family is prone to having kidney stones. Stop use of medicinal quantities of Almonds at least two weeks before a scheduled surgery.[7]

Magical Uses

Almonds and Almond oil are used in spells to attract money, prosperity, beauty, and wisdom. Climb an Almond tree to gain success in business. Almond is an herb of air, and its wood is used to make magic wands. Carry Almonds in your pocket to be guided to treasure.

Almond nuts are sacred to Attis, Mercury, Thoth, and Hermes.[8] Pink flowering Almond trees are sacred to Asherah.

Almonds at Yuletide

Light a menorah and invoke the Goddess Asherah each night, recalling that the original menorah was the image of a flowering Almond, Her sacred tree.

🌙 Marzipan

The almond meal you use to make this marzipan needs to be very dry, so it's probably best to purchase it, rather than make your own from whole almonds.

Makes 6 servings

1½ cups almond meal made from blanched almonds

1½ cups organic confectioners' (powdered) sugar

2 teaspoons pure almond extract

1 teaspoon food-grade rose water

1 free-range organic egg white

Use a food processor to combine the almond flour and confectioners' sugar until there are no lumps.

Add the rose water and almond extract. Pulse.

Add the egg white and pulse again to form a thick dough.

If the mixture is too wet to handle, add more ground almonds and confectioners' sugar and pulse to combine.

Turn the dough out onto a work surface and knead a few times. Form it into a log, wrap it in plastic wrap, and refrigerate for up to 1 month or freeze for up to 6 months.

To use, bring the marzipan to room temperature, then form it into shapes for candy, dip it in chocolate to make truffles, use it to fill a classic stollen, and so on.

Coloring Your Marzipan Creations

Gather your dyes. Use food coloring paste for darker colors or food coloring liquid for lighter colors.

Bring the marzipan to room temperature.

If the dough seems stiff, knead a few drops of corn syrup into it.

Put on some disposable gloves and an apron to protect your clothes.

Use a toothpick to apply a small amount of food coloring, and knead the dough to work it in. Start with just a small amount of coloring; you can always add more if needed.

Shape the colored marzipan as desired, forming animals, vegetables, flowers, et cetera. Use a bit of water, if needed, to smooth out any cracks.

Use a small paintbrush to paint on details such as eyes or flower petals.[9]

Adapted from Kimberly Killebrew's "Best Marzipan and Almond Paste Recipe," Daring Gourmet (website), July 8, 2022.

Apple
(*Malus* spp.)
·················· 🌿 ··················

In medieval Germany, December 24 was called "Adam and Eve Day." The celebration was centered on a "mystery play" or "paradise play," the enactment of the biblical Adam and Eve story for the benefit of the mostly illiterate faithful. At the center of the play was a prop called the Paradise Tree, which was an evergreen, usually a Fir, decorated with Apples to represent the Garden of Eden. Round communion wafers were also hung on the tree to symbolize Jesus and the hope of salvation.

The Paradise Tree merged two mythological trees: the Tree of Life and the Tree of Knowledge of Good and Evil. But it is worth noting that the Bible does not mention Apples. Instead, the European medieval community assumed the enticement of Adam must have occurred by the offer of an Apple. They just couldn't imagine anything more tempting!

Anyway, the play continued to be popular until the fifteenth century, when the Catholic church banned mystery plays altogether. But the Paradise Tree survived by going underground, moving into private homes where families decorated it with Apples and bread wafers. Eventually the wafers were swapped out for cookies, and candles were added for glamour and sparkle.

Another German Christmas tradition was the Christmas Pyramid, a wooden structure decorated with evergreens, figurines, and often a star on top. The Paradise Tree and the Christmas Pyramid eventually morphed into the modern-day Christmas tree. The ornaments that graced the Fir trees, such as Apples and other fruits, cookies, candies and popcorn, glass balls, and figurines, are now fixtures of the Yuletide home decor.[10]

Medicinal Properties
Apples provide fiber, vitamins, minerals, and an array of antioxidants, such as quercetin, catechin, phlorizin, and chlorogenic acid, that help neutralize free radicals (unstable atoms that can damage cells, causing illness and aging). They can provide about 10 percent of our daily vitamin C requirement and 4 percent of our daily potassium requirement.

One study, over the course of 28 years, looked at how consuming

Apples affected the risk of stroke in 9,208 people. It concluded that those who ate the most Apples had a lower risk of thrombotic stroke.[11] Another study found that people who eat the most fiber (like that found in Apples) have a lower risk of cardiovascular disease, coronary heart disease, and stroke.[12]

Eating raw Apples lowers levels of LDL cholesterol levels.[13] Apples appear to help manage blood pressure and can lower the risk of type 2 diabetes. One meta-analysis from 2016 concluded that eating Apples may help lower the risk of lung cancer, breast cancer, and colon cancer, among other types.[14]

Eating raw, peeled Apples can relieve diarrhea and runny stools, while eating baked Apples with the skin still on them can ease constipation. Raw Apple cider can work as a probiotic, helping to replace intestinal flora that may have been killed off by a course of antibiotics.

> **CAUTION: It is worth noting that Apples are loaded with sugars and carbohydrates, so the best Apples for healthy eating are the sour green varieties like Granny Smith. Also, the seeds contain cyanide; eating enough of them (about 1 cup of Apple seeds) could cause death.**

Magical Uses

Like the ancient Celts, you can pour an offering of Apple cider or honey on the ground as thanks when harvesting valuable medicinal plants.

Apples are an herb of love; to attract romance, simmer Apple peels in a large pot or cauldron of water with Cinnamon, Allspice, and/or Ginger. Make a wand of Apple wood to broadcast loving magic, or wear Apple blossom oil to sweeten your love life.

Apples are also associated with immortality and the Summerland; King Arthur's island of Avalon (Abhalloch) was said to be covered with Apples. Make an offering of Apples to the Spirits of your ancestors.

Apples at Yuletide

Decorate your Yule altar and tree with bright red Apples. Cut some round Apple slices and hang them from tree branches as a Solstice offering for the Nature Spirits; cover them in Peanut butter with seeds pressed into it for the birds. Deer and coyotes are quite fond of Apples too; scatter some on the ground as a Yuletide treat.

🍂 Yuletide Potpourri

This brew is not for eating! Use the magical scent to increase love in your home and romance in your life. The apples attract love and the oranges bring joy, the lemons, rosemary, and juniper are purifying, pine bestows peace, ginger inspires energy, and cinnamon gives warmth and protection.

> 2 apples, sliced into rounds
>
> 2 lemons, cut into quarters
>
> 1 orange, sliced into rounds
>
> 3–4 inches fresh ginger, cut into thick coins
>
> 2 large or 4 small cinnamon sticks
>
> 3 long sprigs fresh rosemary
>
> 1 long sprig fresh juniper
>
> 1 long sprig fresh pine
>
> 6 cups water

Combine all the ingredients in a medium pot, cover with the water, and simmer, uncovered, over low heat, or keep on the top of a wood stove. Add more water as the liquid gets low. Allow the aroma to permeate the house.

Adapted from Sandy Coughlin's "Stove-top Yuletide Potpourri Recipe," Reluctant Entertainer (website), December 14, 2018.

🍂 Spiced Apple Cider

This one is for drinking! Here is another magical apple brew that you can actually drink. It has some of the same magical attributes of the potpourri, with allspice for wealth, luck, and healing, nutmeg for success, and cloves to raise spiritual vibrations. Make it with or without bourbon, as desired.

> *Makes 12 servings*

Adapted from Nancy Fuller's "Spiced Cider," FoodNetwork (website), accessed May 22, 2021.

1 gallon organic apple cider

¼ cup organic light brown sugar

1 teaspoon ground allspice

¼ teaspoon ground or grated nutmeg

2 teaspoons whole cloves

1 organic orange

12 cinnamon sticks, one for each serving as a garnish

Bourbon (optional)

Pour the apple cider into a pot and warm over medium heat.

Add the brown sugar, allspice, and nutmeg and stir until the sugar is dissolved. Bring to a low boil.

Stud all the whole cloves into the orange, until just the buds of the cloves are visible. Place the orange in the cider and reduce the heat to maintain a simmer. Cover and simmer for 20 minutes.

Serve warm, with a cinnamon stick garnish in each mug. Add an ounce or two of bourbon to each cup for the grownups.

Bayberry
(*Morella cerifera*)
·················· 🌿 ··················

Bayberries are named after Cape Cod Bay in New England. When the Puritans discovered them, they began making candles with the waxy berries.

Beeswax and Bayberry candles were luxury items in American colonial days. Most candles at that time (used at a rate of about four hundred per year per household) were made of tallow, but tallow candles were smoky and even had an unpleasant smell if they went rancid. Eventually folk traditions developed around the fragrant Bayberry candles.

According to tradition, Bayberry candles may be lit on Winter Solstice Eve, New Year's Eve, or Christmas Eve, after the first star is seen. The lighting of the candles must be timed so they burn until after midnight. If they are burned down to the socket, it's said, a year of prosperity and good fortune will come into the home.

It is also very good luck to give away Bayberry candles. Include a note:

These bayberry candles come from a friend,
So, on Solstice Eve, Christmas Eve, or New Year's Eve,
burn them down to the end,
For a bayberry candle burned to the socket
Will bring joy to the heart and gold to the pocket.

Medicinal Properties

The root bark of Bayberry (also known as Wax Myrtle, Waxberry, or Candleberry) is astringent and has been used to treat digestive disorders such as dysentery, mucus colitis, diarrhea, and looseness or inflammation of the bowels. Female complaints such as uterine prolapse and frequent or heavy periods also fall under its sphere. It is tonic and restorative in fevers and wasting conditions. It is a hot herb and useful for colds and flu.

It can improve digestion in small doses (2 to 5 drops of tincture), while in larger doses (5 to 20 drops) it becomes a gastric stimulant.

A decoction of the root bark may be used as a gargle for sore mouth and throat or in douches and enemas for leukorrhea and fistula. It makes an astringent wash for ulcers, fungal infection of the scalp, and tender, bleeding gums.[15] Bayberry root bark tea can be applied externally as a poultice for cuts, bruises, and wounds.

Native American healers used a decoction of the stems and leaves for fever.

The dosage depends on the preparation:

Decoction: Simmer (do not boil) 1 teaspoon of the root bark, stems, or leaves per cup of water, covered, for 20 minutes. Take up to 2 cups a day, in ¼-cup doses.

Tincture: Take 10 to 30 drops in water four times a day.[16]

> **CAUTION: Bayberry contains high amounts of tannins, which make it useful for binding a loose digestive tract, but it can cause nausea and upset digestion if overused. Bayberry should be avoided by children and in pregnancy and breastfeeding.**

Magical Uses

Bayberry is a New World plant under the expansive dominion of Jupiter. It is used in house blessings, to attract good fortune, to manifest wishes, to bring luck, and to attract money. Carry the dried root in your wallet, scatter it, or burn it as incense. Add a decoction or a few drops of the essential oil to baths and floor washes. Wear the oil to attract a new lover.[17]

Bayberrry at Yuletide

Decorate the house with the fresh boughs of Bayberry at Yuletide. Pinch the leaves to release the scent.

🍂 Bayberry Candles

Bayberries of many species are found on the east and west coasts of the United States, in Europe, and in South America. You can buy, wild-craft, or grow their waxy berries. If wildcrafting, first check to see if bayberry is endangered in your area. Harvest the berries in midfall.

Rinse the berries in a sieve with cold water and place them into a pot. Fill the pot with enough cold water cover the berries by 2 inches. Simmer for an hour. (Don't boil! As with all herbs, boiling drives off the volatile oils, and that is where the scent is.)

Pour off the hot water, saving it and setting it aside; it will contain wax.

Add more cold water to the berries and simmer for another hour. Then pour off the hot water, as before, combining it with the liquid from the first boiling. Compost the boiled berries.

You should see wax floating on the surface of the water. Simmer the water, briefly, so that all the wax floats to the surface. Turn off the heat and let the waxy water cool overnight, or until the wax solidifies. Then remove the wax from the pot.

If you are in the habit of making herbal salves, you will likely have a special pot that you use to melt beeswax. If not, find an old pot and dedicate it to wax melting in the future.

Put the Bayberry wax into your dedicated wax pot. Cover with 3 inches of cold water. Simmer just long enough to melt the wax so you can remove any bits of debris (pieces of twigs, bugs, etc.) that are floating in it. Remove from the heat and allow the wax to solidify again. Dry the wax thoroughly and store it in a cool place.

For candle making, measure out pure beeswax in a 1:2 ratio of beeswax to Bayberry wax, by weight. Measure carefully or the candles will be very brittle.

Add the beeswax and Bayberry wax to your wax pot and set the pot over low heat. Warm until the waxes are melted and combined.

Because beeswax and Bayberry wax burn at different rates, use a wick one size smaller than a wick you'd use for the same size beeswax candle.[18]

Place the wick in the middle of a heat-proof container such as an empty cardboard milk carton or a glass jar. To keep the wick centered you can try wrapping the top of it around a pencil and laying the pencil across the top of the container.

Pour the melted wax into the container then cool the candle for about twenty-four hours, or until completely hardened.

If using a milk carton, peel it away from the wax. If using a jar just leave the wax in the jar.

Birch
(*Betula* spp.)
································ 🌿 ································

In Scotland, the Yule season was once known as "The Yules," and it was an extended celebration including Nollaig Mhòr (Big Christmas, aka Christmas Day) Nollag Bheag (Little Christmas, aka New Year's Day), Hogmanay (First Footing at New Year's), and Oidhche Choinnle (Candle Night), where candles were put in windows to light the way for the Holy Family on Christmas Eve and for First Footers on New Year's Eve.

It was imperative to eat meat after the Sun had set on Yule, because if you didn't, the cattle would suffer in the following year. Traditionally the Yule dishes were cooked over the heat from the Yule Log burning in the hearth throughout the festive season. *Birk* (Birch) was the tree of choice for the Scottish Yule Log, and as long as the Birk log kept burning, the festivities could continue—a good reason to select the largest possible log!

The Yule Log was called the Cailleach Nollich (Old Lady or

Oldwife of Christmas). A female form was chalked onto the log, which would burn away as the fire grew. Was this a memory of keeping death at bay until next Yule by sacrificing a life? A life for a life?

Folk would sit on the Yule Log before it was burned, and even while it was burning, if it was big enough, singing and toasting away. The alcoholic libations may have originally been a way of sanctifying the burning and thanking the tree Spirits for their gifts, such as light, warmth, building materials, food, and medicine.

A piece of the burned Yule Log was kept all year to protect the house from evil sorcery and to draw in luck. It was also reputed to protect the home from fire; a small piece could be tossed into the hearth in the event of a storm to protect the home from lightning. The last piece of the Yule Log left at the end of the year was used to kindle the next year's log.

Birch is also a tree of cleansing and fecundity. In northern Europe, women scourged themselves with Birch twigs in the sauna to increase fertility, while others used it to drive away evil spirits.

Medicinal Properties

Birch inner bark is anti-inflammatory, antibacterial, antifungal, and antiviral. (Always use bark taken from a twig, not the trunk, because taking the bark from the trunk will kill the tree.) It has been used traditionally for bone-related issues such as arthritis and rheumatism, and studies have shown *Betula platyphylla* and *Betula pendula* to be useful in the treatment of degenerative joint disease.

Birch bark is also used for urinary tract issues, gout, and kidney problems. It is chewed to treat sore throat and to lessen excessive menstruation. As a tea, the bark and the sap have been used to treat hepatitis, rash, intestinal worms, and scurvy. Native Americans made extensive use of barks and resins from Birch trees for treating dermatological conditions.

Birch bark also has anticarcinogenic properties; two of its constituents, betulin and betulinic acid, have been extensively studied for this purpose. In vitro, *Betula papyrifera* was found to show cytotoxic activity against human lung carcinoma. All types of Birch barks have shown a pronounced effect against human cancer cell lines.

The leaves and buds of *Betula pubescens* (aka *Betula alba*) have been used for the treatment of cancer of the uterus.

Betula alnoides (Indian Birch, "Tiger Power") is found in East Asia. Its bark is boiled to a gelatinous mass that is applied externally to heal microfractures and bone dislocations in Nepal.[19]

Betula lenta (Black Birch) inner bark is taken for urinary issues and to expel worms. As a decoction, it can be used as a mouthwash and gargle and will help with diarrhea and rheumatic pains.

Betula pubescens (White Birch) leaf tea, taken daily, helps with gravel and stone in the kidneys. For treating skin conditions, it is used externally as a wash or is added to bathwater.

To make an infusion of the leaves: Steep 2 tablespoons of crushed leaves per cup freshly boiled water, covered, for about 20 minutes. Take up to 1½ cups per day in very small doses. The leaves have to be fresh, and they are best gathered before Summer Solstice (freeze them for later use if necessary).

To make a decoction of the bark: Simmer 1 teaspoon of bark per cup of water for 20 minutes in a tightly covered, nonaluminum pan. Take up to 2 cups a day in ½-teaspoon doses.[20]

All Birches except White Birch have a lovely wintergreen flavor and smell, and the inner bark can be prepared as a beverage tea. The tea is mildly sedative and will help you sleep. I like to gather the fresh inner bark of Black Birch, Yellow Birch, or River Birch (anything except White Birch, which has no scent) in the spring when the sap is rising in the trees. I use the inner bark in soothing medicinal salves and combine it with Sassafras root bark and Ginger root in teas.

CAUTION: Birch pollen can be an irritant for people who are sensitive to Wild Carrot, Mugwort, Apples, Soybeans, Hazelnuts, and Peanuts. Birch leaf may cause sodium retention and worsen high blood pressure. Do not use Birch with "water pills" (diuretics), as it could cause excessive water loss and a drop in blood pressure.[21]

Magical Uses

Birch is one of the first trees to colonize an area that has been denuded of trees, and for this reason it is sometimes called the "tree of new beginnings." Its name is also the first letter (*beith*) of the ancient Celtic ogham alphabet. Write your petition on a scrap of Birch bark and give it to the fire; the smoke will carry your wishes to the Gods. A traditional Witch's *besom* (broom) is made from Birch twigs with an Ash handle and Willow bindings.

Birch at Yuletide

Find a large Birch log and burn it at Yule. For those who do not have a fireplace, drill three holes into a Birch log and place a candle into each hole. At Winter Solstice, burn one candle for the ancestors, one for the Nature Spirits, and one for the Gods.

Birch Bark Is Edible

Birch bark (and also Pine bark) was once a staple food for many indigenous peoples. The inner bark was ground for use as a type of flour, especially by the Sami people in northern Sweden, who mixed the ground bark with reindeer milk to make bread. In Russia, it was once mixed with rye flour to make rye bread.

Look for the inner bark, the reddish layer between the distinctive papery outer bark and inner hardwood, which is dead. The inner bark can be gathered from any Birch tree that is not dormant, frozen, or rotten from having fallen down a while ago. It has the best flavor in spring and early summer. Ethically, bark should be taken only from the trunk of a tree that has recently fallen or is about to be cut, because stripping bark from the trunk will kill the tree. A better solution is to find a twig or small branch and strip the bark from that.

Once you have stripped the thin, living layer of inner bark from the outer bark, dry it. You might place the curls of inner bark in a dehydrator, near a wood stove, or in the oven at 250°F for 30 minutes.

Once the bark is dry, grind it coarsely with a food processor, then finish with a mortar and pestle or a coffee grinder (I have a coffee grinder that I use only for herbs, acorns, and the like). You might want to sift the resulting flour after that, to make sure no large particles remain.

🍂 Birch Bark Cookies

> ¾ cup organic white flour (or wheat flour substitute, like
> rice flour), plus a bit for flouring your work surface
> ¼ cup birch bark flour
> ¼ cup organic sugar
> Pinch of sea salt
> ½ cup organic butter, at room temperature

Preheat the oven to 350°F.

Combine the white flour, birch bark flour, sugar, and salt in a large bowl and mix well. Add the butter and blend until it's well mixed. Knead briefly.

Roll out the dough on a floured surface to make a large flat pancake, and cut out cookie shapes (use cookie cutters or an upside-down glass). Lay the cookie shapes on a baking sheet. Bake for about 15 minutes.

Adapted from Ashley Adamant's "How to Make Birch Bark Flour (Plus Birch Shortbread Cookies," Practical Self Reliance (website), April 26, 2018.

Boxwood
(*Buxus sempervirens*)

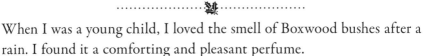

When I was a young child, I loved the smell of Boxwood bushes after a rain. I found it a comforting and pleasant perfume.

In Europe in the Middle Ages, Boxwood wood was prized for making fine objects such as writing tablets, figurines, spice boxes, prayer beads, and reliquaries to hold holy water. It became even more popular when the ivory trade was disrupted by the Ottoman Turks. Fragrant Boxwood even had a biblical imprimatur:

The glory of Lebanon shall come unto thee, the fir tree,
the pine tree, and the box together, to beautify the place
of my sanctuary; and I will make the place of my feet
glorious.

ISAIAH 60:13

In the twelfth century, Boxwood and Laurel were sanctioned, along with Palms, for the Palm Sunday processions. An herb of protection, Boxwood even had a reputation for driving out the Devil.[22] (Who says Christians don't believe in magic?)

Here is a sort of herbal calendar from the seventeenth century, defined by the putting up and taking down of greenery:

Down with rosemary and bays,
Down with the mistletoe;
Instead of holly, now up-raise
The greener box, for show.

The holly hitherto did sway;
Let Box now domineer,
Until the dancing Easter-day,
Or Easter's eve appear.

Then youthful box, which now hath grace
Your houses to renew,
Grown old, surrender must his place
Unto the crisped yew.

When yew is out, then birch comes in,
And many flowers beside,
Both of a fresh and fragrant kin,
To honour Whitsuntide.

Green rushes then, and sweetest bents,
With cooler oaken boughs,

> *Come in for comely ornaments*
> *To re-adorn the house.*
> *Thus times do shift; each thing his turn does hold,*
> *New things succeed, as former things grow old.*
> ROBERT HERRICK, "CEREMONIES FOR CANDLEMAS
> EVE" (SEVENTEENTH CENTURY)

Medicinal Properties

Boxwood leaves are collected in the spring (before the Summer Solstice) and can be dried for later use. The bark also is dried before use. Boxwood leaves and bark have been used for malaria, gout, rheumatism, urinary tract infections, intestinal worms, chronic skin problems, syphilis, and hemorrhoids.

Boxwood is diaphoretic (causes sweating) and purgative (flushes the bowels).

CAUTION: This plant can kill livestock. It should not be used except with caution and under the supervision of a trained herbalist or naturopath. The side effects can include abdominal pain, vomiting, bloody diarrhea, tremors, loss of coordination, convulsions, dizziness, coma, and even death due to respiratory paralysis.[23]

Magical Uses

Boxwood is slow-growing and evergreen, making it an herb of longevity, stability, stoicism, and immortality. The Greeks considered Boxwood to be sacred to Pluto, protector of all evergreens, and symbolic of the life that continues through winter in the Underworld.[24] It is also connected to Athena, who has a flute carved from Boxwood.

Because it persists and thrives in difficult circumstances, Boxwood is an herb of protection and comfort. Use it to make an amulet for protection from evil forces.[25]

Boxwood at Yuletide

Because it is an evergreen, Boxwood is a classic herb of immortality and suitable for winter rites of all kinds. It's biblical associations noted above make it doubly apt for this season. Place a boxwood carved figurine amid your Christmas decorations or create a Boxwood Yuletide tree. Two of these trees would look nice on either side of an altar, dedicated to the Gods of the Underworld, or just make one as a tabletop centerpiece.

🌱 A Boxwood Yuletide Tree

Floral foam block, to stick the stems into (available at craft stores)

Knife, for carving the floral foam

Shears or sturdy scissors, to cut stems

A waterproof container (a vase, mug, wooden box lined with plastic), to hold the floral foam block

Boxwood branches, cut about 6 inches long

Rose bush branches or branches with red berries, cut about 6 inches long

Long-stemmed red roses, cut about 6 inches long (if you feel like splurging)

Soak the floral foam block in water. Then place it into your container. It should fit snugly.

Use a knife to sculpt your block, rounding it into a vague cone shape that is gently pointed at the top and slopes out to the full width of the container at the point where it meets that container.

Push the base of one boxwood branch into the point of the floral foam cone.

Add branches at the bottom and all the way around the floral foam block until you form a "tree" that appears bushy and symmetrical. Place your rose branches, berry branches, or roses stems at natural intervals around the tree.

Water the "tree" every other day so the block stays wet and the "tree" looks green and healthy for 2 to 3 weeks.

Adapted from Fine Gardening's "How to Make a Holiday Boxwood Tree," on the Fine Gardening website, accessed May 30, 2021.

Cacao
(*Theobroma cacao*)

Cacao was used as a ceremonial medicine as far back as 1500 BCE by the Olmecs, the earliest recorded civilization in Mexico, and was later adopted and used by both the Aztec and Mayan cultures. According to legend, Moctezuma II, ruler of the Aztec Empire, introduced Cacao to the Spanish conquistador Hernán Cortés.

Theobroma is Greek for "food of the Gods" (*theos* meaning "God," and *broma* meaning "food"). The word *cacao* comes from the Nahuatl name for this plant, *cacahuatl*. The ancient Mayans believed that the Gods first discovered Cacao on a sacred mountain. They fermented and dried the beans, roasted them, and ground them into paste. The paste was mixed with water, cornmeal, Chili peppers, and other spices, then poured back and forth between two containers until frothy. Nobles and clergy (and, on special occasions, commoners) would sip the beverage as a fine digestif after a meal.

Cacao also featured in religious rituals honoring the Mayan Gods; the liquid chocolate could at times stand in for blood. Ek Chuaj (also known as Ek Chuah or Ekchuah) was the God of Cacao. Cacao beans and utensils for preparing chocolate were deposited in the tombs of deceased rulers, while brides and grooms drank the sacred beverage during their marriage rite. In baptisms, babies were anointed with ground Cacao beans mixed with ground up flowers and pure water from tree hollows.

The Aztecs learned to use Cacao from the Mayans. Unable to grow the trees in arid Mexico, they demanded the beans as tribute from conquered peoples and formed trade routes just to obtain the beans. The Aztecs were very strict about who had access to the sacred drink; only nobles, clergy, great warriors, prominent merchants, and honored guests were allowed to partake of it, and it was said to bestow power and wisdom. The beans were more valuable than gold or silver and eventually became a form of currency.

Aztec religion held that they had received Cacao from the God Quetzalcoatl, who came down from the heavens on the beam of a morning star bearing a Cacao tree from paradise. The Aztecs, in turn, made offerings of Cacao to their Gods and used *cacahuatl* (cacao water) as a ritual drink.[26]

Medicinal Properties

Both cocoa and chocolate are derived from Cacao. Cocoa ranks high among foods with the highest antioxidant polyphenol content. It has been shown to reduce blood pressure and provides great cardio-protection. It also stimulates the production of serotonin and dopamine, making it antidepressant and mood-elevating.[27]

Cocoa is used for infectious intestinal diseases, diarrhea, asthma, and bronchitis and as an expectorant for lung congestion. It can be beneficial for liver, bladder, and kidney ailments and as a general health tonic.

Early research indicates that cocoa may be helpful for chronic fatigue syndrome, as well as the anxiety and depression that accompany that condition. Cocoa may improve liver function and help with cirrhosis (liver disease resulting from viral hepatitis or from alcohol consumption).

The husks of the cacao seed may help with constipation, including in children.

Milk chocolate also comes from Cacao beans but chocolate candy is only about ten percent cocoa on average and milk chocolate often has a lot of sugar, which is not ideal for human health. For health benefits look for dark chocolate that is more than 70 percent cocoa to maximize the antioxidant effect. For high blood pressure, try 46 to 105 grams of dark chocolate per day, providing 213 to 500 milligrams of polyphenols.[28]

CAUTION: Cocoa contains caffeine, which can increase anxiety, urination, sleeplessness, and irregular heartbeat and worsen glaucoma, osteoporosis, and IBS. In some individuals it can produce a rash, constipation, migraine headaches, nausea, intestinal discomfort, or gas. Persons with bleeding disorders should avoid it as it slows blood clotting. Cocoa can worsen GERD and can increase blood sugar levels in diabetics.

> Women who are pregnant or breastfeeding should consume cocoa only in food amounts (less than 200 milligrams daily). High doses of caffeine are thought to potentially result in premature delivery, low birth weight, and miscarriage. Caffeine passes through a mother's breast milk and can cause irritability and loose bowels in a nursing baby.
>
> Stop eating cocoa at least 2 weeks before a scheduled surgery due to its blood-thinning action.[29]

Magical Uses

Use chocolate in rituals to strengthen bonds of love between celebrants and all creatures of the Earth. Drink it to empower a guided meditation or trance journey. Make an offering of the drink and drink it to commune with deities, especially Aztec, Mayan, Olmec, and other Mesoamerican Gods and Goddesses. Consume Cacao to navigate through your personal pain to an awareness of your own divinity.

Eat or drink chocolate, or share it in ritual, to increase feelings of camaraderie, love, self-love, and nurturing of self and others or just for fun. Giving and receiving chocolate makes a romance blossom. Eating chocolate attracts happiness and prosperity.

Cacao at Yuletide

When invoking or making an offering to a Mesoamerican God or Goddess, why not serve up a traditional Mexican chocolate drink? After all, this is what the Gods have come to expect. Cacao and chocolate are an appropriate offering to the Mesoamerican Solar deities at the time of the Winter Solstice.

Kinich Ahau (Sun-Faced Ruler) is the Sun God of the Mayans, associated with kings and nobles. Huitzilopochtli is the Aztec God of war, the Sun, and sacrifice. Tonatiuh (Nahuatl: "Movement of the Sun") is an Aztec Sun God of the daytime sky who rules the cardinal direction of east. Inti is the ancient Incan Sun God.

Other solar deities may also enjoy being honored with chocolate. Ra is an Egyptian God of the Sun and creator God. The Germanic Sol, Vedic Surya, and Greek Helios (Apollo) are also solar deities. In the days of the Roman Empire, the festival of the birth of the Unconquered Sun (Dies Natalis Solis Invicti) was observed on the Winter Solstice—December 25 of the Julian calendar. The religious celebrations on December 25 were eventually replaced with the observance of the birthday of Jesus Christ (Christmas).

A number of Egyptian Goddesses are also associated with the Sun: Wadjet, Sekhmet, Hathor, Nut, Bast, Bat, and Menhit. Isis gave birth to Horus, the Egyptian God whose body represents the heavens and whose eyes represent the Sun and Moon, and both Isis and Hathor nursed him.

Among the Greeks, Alectrona (Electryone or Electryo) is the Goddess of the Sun, while Artemis, twin sister of Apollo, is Goddess of the Sun and Moon. Sunna is the Norse Sun Goddess, while Amaterasu is the Japanese Shinto Sun Goddess. Áine is the Irish Goddess of the summer Sun and Grainne, her sister, is the Goddess of the fainter winter Sun.

There are many other solar deities. Find one that calls to you at Solstice, and pour out an offering of sweet chocolate in their honor. Below are two traditional Mexican chocolate libations to get you started.

For these drinks, you will ideally use *chocolate de metate* (stone-ground chocolate), flavored with sugar and cinnamon (find it in your grocery store or order it online). The chocolate is melted and then whipped to a froth using a *molinillo* (wooden whisk), but a wire whisk will work if that's what you have on hand. The drinks should be light and very frothy when served.

🌿 Chocolate Caliente Mexicano (Mexican Hot Chocolate)

You can make the chocolate with water or milk; water will yield a stronger cacao flavor, while milk will yield a richer drink. Both are traditional.

Makes 4 servings

> 6 ounces organic Mexican chocolate
> 4¼ cups organic milk or water
> 4 cinnamon sticks, for garnish

Adapted from Douglas Cullen's "Mexican Hot Chocolate," Mexican Food Journal (website), accessed June 2, 2021.

Pour the milk or water into a pot and set it over very low heat. Warm the milk, but do not allow it to boil.

Once bubbles start appearing in the milk, add the chocolate. When it begins to dissolve, stir the mixture with a *molinillo* (or whisk). Continue warming, stirring the mixture steadily, until the chocolate fully dissolves, about 20 minutes.

If the milk comes close to boiling, remove the pot from the heat for a couple of minutes, while continuing to stir, and after a few minutes return the pot to the heat.

Once the chocolate has fully dissolved, vigorously froth the drink with the *molinillo* (or whisk) until it develops a foamy, creamy texture, about 10 minutes.

Serve warm, garnished with a cinnamon stick floating in each mug.

🍂 Chocolate Caliente con Kahlua (Mexican Hot Chocolate with Kahlua)

Makes 2 servings

> 3 cups organic whole milk
> 3 ounces organic Mexican chocolate
> 2 cinnamon sticks
> 6 tablespoons Kahlua or coffee liqueur

Place the milk and cinnamon sticks in a pan and set it over very low heat. Warm the milk, but do not allow it to boil.

Once bubbles start appearing in the milk, add the chocolate. When it begins to dissolve, stir the mixture with a *molinillo* (or whisk). Continue warming, stirring, and frothing until the chocolate fully dissolves, about 20 minutes.

Once the chocolate has fully dissolved, add the Kahlua and froth again with the *molinillo* (or whisk) for a few seconds. Serve immediately.

Adapted from Andrés Carnalla's "Mexican Kahlua Hot Chocolate," Mexican Food Journal (website), accessed June 2, 2021.

Cinnamon
(Cinnamomum cassia, Cinnamomum verum)

·················· 🌿 ··················

A garden enclosed
Is my sister, my spouse,
A spring shut up,
A fountain sealed.
Your plants are an orchard of pomegranates
With pleasant fruits,
Fragrant henna with spikenard,
Spikenard and saffron,
Calamus and cinnamon,
With all trees of frankincense,
Myrrh and aloes,
With all the chief spices—
A fountain of gardens,
A well of living waters,
And streams from Lebanon.

SONG OF SOLOMON 4:12–15

Cinnamon spice comes from the inner bark of trees in the *Cinnamomum* genus; Cinnamon from *Cinnamomum cassia* is stronger and spicier, while that from *Cinnamomum verum*, sometimes called "true Cinnamon," which comes originally from Sri Lanka (Ceylon), is sweeter. Other types of Cinnamon are on the market and all can be used interchangeably in cooking.

Long before it became known in Europe, the Egyptians, Greeks, Romans, and Chinese used Cinnamon in their cooking and as medicine. The ancient Egyptians employed it in the embalming process, and in the first century CE, Pliny the Elder wrote that it was fifteen times more valuable than silver by weight. In the Middle Ages people used Cinnamon to preserve meat and to mask the odor of rotting flesh.

By the fifteenth century, Cinnamon was more valuable than gold, and it was one of the spurs to European exploration and colonization of the world. It is native to southwest Asia, but its true source was long a jealously guarded secret. A mythology arose around its origin: giant cinnamologus birds from Arabia were said to collect Cinnamon sticks from an unknown place where the trees flourished and use the fragrant sticks to build their nests. The sticks were harvested by a process that required dislodging the birds from their cliff-hanging nests by various heroic measures.

Cinnamon had holy connotations in the ancient world: It was a sacred plant of Dionysus, the Greek God of ecstasy. The phoenix, which died and was reborn from its ashes in mythology, was said to use Cinnamon, Myrrh, and Spikenard to build the magic fire in which it was reincarnated. The Chinese burned Cinnamon in their temples, as did the ancient Greeks as an offering to the Gods. The Roman emperor Nero is said to have ordered a year's supply of Cinnamon be burned at his wife's funeral as penance after he murdered her.[30]

Cinnamon has a long history of colonial exploitation. The spice trade was monopolized by royalty; kings entered into contracts with foreign merchants, fixed the prices, and received the revenue. The people of the land where the trees grew were not involved, nor did they benefit from the trade.

When the Portuguese took control of Sri Lanka (Ceylon) in the 1500s, they also took over the island's Cinnamon production and commerce. Dutch traders displaced the Portuguese by 1640, and when the Dutch learned of another source of Cinnamon along the coast of India, they bribed and threatened the local king to destroy it, thus preserving their monopoly. Then the French seized Sri Lanka from the Dutch, and in 1795 England seized it from the French. But by 1833, a number of other tropical countries had begun producing Cinnamon and the monopoly was finally broken.[31]

Medicinal Properties

References to the medicinal uses of Cinnamon date as far back as ancient Chinese texts of 2800 BCE. Both *Cinnamomum cassia* and *Cinnamomum verum* are used in medicine.

Indian Ayurvedic medicine uses Cinnamon as a remedy for respiratory, digestive, and gynecological complaints. "True Cinnamon"

(*Cinnamomum verum*) has anti-inflammatory and antimicrobial properties, reduces cardiovascular disease, boosts cognitive function, and lowers the risk of colon cancer. It has been shown to increase circulating insulin levels in diabetics and has beneficial effects against diabetic neuropathy (numbness or weakness in peripheral nerves) and nephropathy (kidney disease cause by diabetes). It also helps lower blood glucose, serum cholesterol, and blood pressure, leading to beneficial cardiovascular effects.

Cinnamon has high levels of antioxidants (meaning that it is protective against free radicals, which may play a role in heart disease, cancer, and other diseases) and may be protective against Alzheimer's disease.

Thanks to its warming nature, Cinnamon tea can help with menstrual cramping and pain, coughing, and bronchitis and other chest complaints. It also is antidiarrheal and can help heal gastric ulcers.

Added to salves and ointments, Cinnamon speeds skin healing.[32]

To prepare it as a tea, simmer 1 small stick or 1 teaspoon ground Cinnamon per cup of water in a nonaluminum pot with a tight lid for 15 to 20 minutes. Drink in ¼-cup doses.

One half teaspoon to one teaspoon can be taken daily on Oatmeal or in tea to lower A1C levels.[33]

> **CAUTION: Avoid Cinnamon if you are allergic to it, of course, and also if you are allergic to Balsam of Peru (*Myroxylon balsamum*). Do not combine it with other drugs that may be toxic to the liver. Pregnant and breastfeeding women can use it safely in food amounts but should avoid medicinal amounts.**

Magical Uses

Cinnamon is an herb of protection; hang bunches of Cinnamon sticks over entrances and place the sticks along windowsills. Burn it to repel negative energies, carry it on your person, or simmer it on the stove to fill your home with the comforting and protective scent.

Serve the tea, burn the spice, or add it to a love potion to heat up a romance.

Put a piece of the bark or a few drops of the essential oil into your wallet, or burn it at your place of business to attract money.

Cinnamon at Yuletide

Hot, spicy Cinnamon is a classic Christmas spice. Burn it as incense on the altar at Winter Solstice and serve it in cakes, cookies, and drinks after a ritual or during a holiday party.

🍂 Bourbon Eggnog

Kitchen Witches and Hearth Druids will appreciate this spicy blend of nutmeg, which increases insight, clarity, and mental concentration; cinnamon, which brings in protection, love, and abundance; allspice, for healing and plenty; and clove, which fosters protection, healing, and wealth. The eggs and milk hold the energies of the Great Mother who nourishes us all.

Make this drink the day before your event so all the flavors have a chance to settle.

Makes 8 servings

> 4 free-range organic eggs
> ¾ cup organic sugar
> 1 teaspoon freshly grated nutmeg
> ½ teaspoon ground cinnamon
> ⅛ teaspoon ground allspice
> ⅛ teaspoon ground cloves
> 8 tablespoons bourbon
> 4 tablespoons cognac
> 4 tablespoons brandy-based orange liqueur, such as
>   Cointreau
> 1½ cups organic whole milk
> 1 cup organic heavy cream
> Grated nutmeg or ground cinnamon, for garnish

Blend the eggs in a mixer or a blender for 1 minute. Add the sugar, nutmeg, cinnamon, allspice, and cloves and blend for 30 seconds. Add the bourbon,

Adapted from Colleen Graham's "Bourbon Eggnog," The Spruce Eats (website), accessed June 7, 2021.

cognac, and orange liqueur and blend for another 30 seconds. Add the milk and cream and blend for 1 minute.

Pour the eggnog into another container, cover it, and refrigerate. Let steep in the refrigerator for a day.

When serving, grate fresh nutmeg or cinnamon over the top, if you like.

A Note about Using Raw Eggs

Buy only good-quality, organic eggs that have been kept continuously refrigerated and have no cracks. Always check the sell-by date on the carton.

Refrigerate your eggs in the coldest part of the refrigerator (do not store them in the refrigerator door). Do not store eggs for more than 3 weeks.

Test your eggs by floating them in water. If they sink, they are fine. If they float, they are no longer edible.

When you crack an egg, if any part looks cloudy or otherwise off, don't use it.

Clove
(Syzygium aromaticum)
·················· 🦌 ··················

Cloves are the dried flower buds of a tropical evergreen tree native to the Maluku Islands (the Spice Islands) of Indonesia. Their name comes from the Latin *clavus* (nail).

Cloves were a much desired spice during the Middle Ages, used to flavor and preserve food. The prohibitive cost and rarity of the spice may have been one reason it was used for the high holy day of Christmas. The cost of importing Cloves was once so high that they were as valuable as gold, and trade wars were fought over them. The Dutch even destroyed trees they found that were growing in areas outside their control.

Cloves were sacred to the indigenous peoples of the Spice Islands. Natives of the area would plant a Clove tree when a child was born.

The growth and health of the tree was said to predict the course of the child's life.[34]

Medicinal Properties

Cloves are antioxidant, hepatoprotective, antimicrobial, and anti-inflammatory. They can improve digestion and control gastrointestinal irritation. As antibacterials, they are helpful in wound salves and creams. They are protective for the liver and can help control blood sugar levels. They increase the white blood cell count, thus boosting immunity. Cloves (and Nutmeg!) have also shown aphrodisiac properties.

Clove extracts help reduce gum diseases such as gingivitis and periodontitis, and diluted Clove oil is applied to the gums to ease the pain of toothache, though it may cause irritation in some individuals (call your dentist!).

A few drops of the essential oil taken in water can stop vomiting and relieve nausea.

> **CAUTION: Never apply Clove essential oil directly to the skin or gums. Dilute it first with a carrier oil, such as Olive. Contrary to myth, Clove cigarettes are not "healthy"; they actually contain more nicotine, carbon monoxide, and tar than tobacco cigarettes.[35] Do not give Clove oil to children by mouth; it is too irritating for them. Clove is safe in food amounts for pregnant and breastfeeding women but should be avoided in medicinal amounts. Avoid Clove if you have a bleeding disorder and for 2 weeks before a scheduled surgery, as it can slow blood clotting. Do not take Clove in combination with other anticoagulants.[36]**

Magical Uses

Cloves are herbs of protection that also attract prosperity, while Oranges (*Citrus sinensis*) are solar fruits with the joyful, expansive, positive energy of our nearest star. Clove-studded Orange pomanders are natural charms for protection and good luck that can be kept for years when carefully dried.

Cloves at Yuletide

The bright color of the solar Oranges and the scent of protective Clove enliven your home at Yule.

🍂 Clove-Studded Orange Pomander

To make pomanders, prick ripe Oranges with a toothpick or other sharp instrument to make spirals, pentagrams, whorls, or other patterns on the skin. Then stud the Oranges with the dried Clove buds, placing one Clove into each hole you pricked. (You will need 1 to 2 ounces of Cloves per Orange, so buy them in bulk.)

Keep the finished pomanders on display in a bowl, hang them in bathrooms and closets, or place them in drawers. Suspend them in the kitchen near where fresh fruits and vegetables are stored to repel insects.[37]

To hang the pomanders, drive a wire straight through each Orange, and form both ends of the wire, at the top and the bottom of the pomander, into a small loop. You can then thread a colorful ribbon through the top loop or hang other magical herbs from the bottom loop.

To dry the pomanders, you can coat them with a natural preservative spice mixture and let them air-dry (see below).[38] Alternatively, if you have a dehydrator, use it to dry the pomanders at medium heat (105°F to 115°F) until they are hard. Or bake them in a low oven (105°F to 115°F) until they are dry and hard.

Preservative Spice Blend for Drying Pomanders

¾ cup powdered orris root

½ cup ground cinnamon

¼ cup ground cloves

2 tablespoons ground ginger

2 tablespoons ground nutmeg

Combine these ground spices and store them in a jar or other airtight container until you are ready to use them.

To use, pour the mixture into a paper bag, drop in the pomanders, and shake to coat them thoroughly. Leave them in the bag of spices for 2 to 6 weeks to prevent mold growth as they dry.

🍂 Spicy Glazed Winter Solstice Scones

Kitchen Witches and Hearth Druids take note: With cinnamon for power, luck, and lust, nutmeg for prosperity and clear thinking, clove for protection, healing, and abundance, ginger for love and to heat up and amplify the action of all spells, and pumpkin for love, prosperity, and fertility, these scones will empower your Christmas wishes and Yuletide dreams. Serve them with mulled wine or spiced apple cider during or after your Solstice rite.

Makes 10 scones

> 2 cups organic flour
> ⅓ cup organic sugar
> 1 tablespoon aluminum-free baking powder
> ½ teaspoon sea salt
> 1 teaspoon ground cinnamon
> ½ teaspoon ground nutmeg
> ¼ teaspoon ground cloves
> ¼ teaspoon ground ginger
> 6 tablespoons organic butter, cut into small pieces
> ½ cup organic pumpkin puree (not canned pumpkin pie filling)
> 3 tablespoons organic milk (or milk substitute, such as rice, almond, or oat milk)
> 1 free-range organic egg

> For the Glaze
> 1 cup plus 3 tablespoons organic confectioners' (powdered) sugar
> 2 tablespoons organic milk (or milk substitute such as rice, almond, oat milk, etc.)
> ¼ teaspoon ground cinnamon
> Pinch of ground nutmeg
> Pinch of ground cloves
> Pinch of ground ginger

Preheat the oven to 425°F. Line a baking sheet with parchment paper. (You do

---

Adapted from Linda Lum's "Pumpkin Spice Scones," a recipe in "Exploring Cloves: The Christmas Spice Adds a Touch of Heat to Every Meal," Delishably (website), November 24, 2022.

not need to put any grease or oil on the parchment paper, and it can be used for several batches of the same recipe.)

In a large bowl, whisk together the flour, sugar, baking powder, salt, cinnamon, nutmeg, cloves, and ginger. Using a pastry blender (or food processor), cut in the butter until the mixture resembles coarse sand.

In a separate bowl, whisk together the pumpkin, milk, and egg.

Add the pumpkin mixture to the dry ingredients. Mix briefly.

Pat out the dough on a lightly floured surface to form a rectangle that is roughly 4 inches by 12 inches. Cut the dough into thirds to form three 4-inch by 4-inch squares. Cut an X through each square to form four triangular scones.

Place the scones on the lined baking sheet and bake for 14 to 16 minutes, or until lightly browned on the bottom. Remove from the oven and let cool.

While the scones are cooling, make the glaze: Whisk together the confectioners' sugar, milk, and spices. Drizzle the spiced glaze over the scones.

Cranberry
(Vaccinium macrocarpon)
······················ 🍁 ······················

Bright red berries that are native to and grown only in North America, Cranberries are harvested from bogs in late autumn, which may be a reason they became associated with late fall and winter festivals such as Thanksgiving and Christmas.

Native Americans used the berries as a dye for clothing and blankets, as a healing agent, and as food. The Pequot of Cape Cod called the berry *ibimi* (bitter berry). Mashed Cranberries were combined with venison and fat to make pemmican (a paste of dried and pounded meat mixed with melted fat and berries), and the berries were applied as poultices to draw poison from arrow wounds. Native Americans taught English settlers how to use the berries, and they may well have been included in the first Thanksgiving feast.[39]

The Lenni Lenape people have a story that carries the tribal memory of struggles with ancient mastodons. According to the legend, the mastodon was a beast of burden for all the animals but grew tired of that task and longed to be the king of all creatures. Eventually, a great battle took place between the animals. The fighting was so intense that the Great Spirit had to step in to stop the carnage, and lightning bolts rained down from the heavens, causing the land to churn into a bog. Then Great Spirit covered the blasted devastation with green vines that blossomed into pink flowers and finally bore bright red fruits. Ever after, the Cranberry was known as the symbol of peace.

The great sachem (chief) of the Delaware was called Pakimintzen (Cranberry Eater). He ate cranberries at peace festivals as a symbol of lasting order and goodwill.[40] For many of the First Nations, the berries' color—red—is associated with the "good red road" (the right path of life), and a person associated with the color red is someone who lives a life of wisdom and integrity.

Cranberries are often strung alone or with white popcorn to make garlands for Christmas trees, a fitting symbol for the season of "peace on Earth."

Medicinal Properties

For medicinal purposes, it's best to use fresh Cranberries and pure, unsweetened Cranberry juice. Cranberries provide fiber, vitamin C, flavonoids, phenols, and other substances that can help with urinary tract infections, cancer, heart disease, and other chronic conditions. Cranberries even contain a chemical that blocks pathogens that cause tooth decay.[41]

Cranberry juice binds with *E. coli* bacteria in the urinary tract, blocking the bacteria's ability to adhere to the urinary tract wall. Taken daily (diluted with water), it can prevent urinary tract infections.[42]

A cranberry compress or poultice made with the crushed fruits in cheesecloth can be applied externally to help heal hemorrhoids and fistulas.

Taking 120 to 800 milligrams of dried Cranberry, in capsules or tablets, once or twice daily has shown success for preventing urinary tract infections (UTIs) in adults. Or you could drink ¼ cup of unsweetened Cranberry juice four times a day, between meals.

Children can take ¼ cup of a Cranberry and Lingonberry (*Vaccinium vitis-idaea*) concentrate or unsweetened cranberry juice daily for 6 months. One study used 120 milligrams of a standardized Cranberry extract (Anthocran) daily for 60 days in children 12 to 18 years of age.[43]

> CAUTION: Drinking too much Cranberry juice could cause mild stomach upset and diarrhea and may increase the risk of kidney stones in individuals who are vulnerable. Those who are pregnant or breastfeeding and those with an allergy to aspirin should probably avoid Cranberries. Cranberry juices act as a mild blood thinner. Use caution when taking medicinal doses of Cranberry in combination with other blood thinners such as warfarin or aspirin.[44]

Magical Uses

You can use Cranberry juice in place of wine in rituals. Red foods and juices are associated with the heart, so use Cranberries in brews to engender love. You can also place them on the harvest altar in thanks for the work of the Devas and Land Spirits who helped create the crops we eat.

Cranberries are sacred to Mars and to Astarte/Ashtoreth, Queen of Heaven and Goddess of sex and love, to whom the Canaanites once burned offerings and poured libations (Jeremiah 44).

Cranberries at Yuletide

Add Cinnamon and Clove to your Cranberry sauce and eat it to bring energy to your projects. Serve a Cranberry drink or food to your loved one. String the fresh berries into garlands (maybe with some popcorn added!) for your Yule tree.

To increase your attitude of gratitude as the dark days of winter creep in, put eight ripe cranberries into a bowl. Place the bowl on your seasonal altar, and every day pick up the berries, one at a time. For each berry you pick up, say one thing you are grateful for, then put the berries back into the bowl.

🍃 Cranberry Yuletide Punch

A perfect libation for your Winter Solstice soiree. Kitchen Witches and Hearth Druids will appreciate the energizing influence of Mars and the deep spirituality of Astarte, courtesy of the cranberries, complemented by limes for purification in the coming year and oranges and lemons for their solar influence.

Regular ice cubes will dilute the flavor when they melt. For best results, use cranberry juice ice cubes, freezing the juice in an ice cube tray. You can make an alcohol-free version for kids.

Makes 10 servings

> 4 cups organic unsweetened cranberry juice
> 1 cup organic orange juice
> 1 cup tequila
> 1 cup vodka
> ½ cup triple sec
> Sweetener (organic sugar, maple syrup or maple sugar, or stevia), if needed
> 2¼ cups (10 ounces) organic cranberries, frozen
> 2 organic oranges, sliced thin
> 2 organic limes, sliced thin
> 1 organic lemon, sliced thin
> Organic cranberry juice ice cubes
> Club soda

Pour the cranberry juice, orange juice, tequila, vodka, and triple sec into a large punch bowl. Stir gently. Taste the blend, and if it seems too bitter, add a bit of sweetener.

Float the citrus slices in the blend. Add the frozen cranberries and enough cranberry ice to chill everything well (add more cranberry ice later, as needed).

Serve in punch glasses, with a splash of club soda added to each portion.

Adapted from Macheesmo's "Cranberry Moonshine Punch," Tablespoon (website), November 5, 2019.

Frankincense and Myrrh
(*Boswellia sacra*) and (*Commiphora myrrha*)

.... 🌿 ....

*And when they were come into the house, they saw
the young child with Mary his mother, and fell down,
and worshipped him: and when they had opened their
treasures, they presented unto him gifts; gold, and
frankincense and myrrh.*

MATTHEW 2:11

Frankincense comes from the northern and western regions of Africa,
as well as the southern deserts of Oman and Yemen and India. Myrrh
is native to northeastern Africa, as well as Oman, Yemen, and parts of
Saudi Arabia. But the resinous Burseraceae family, which includes both
Frankincense and Myrrh, originally evolved in the region we now know
as Mexico during the Paleocene era (about sixty-five million years ago),
before the continents drifted apart.

Frankincense and Myrrh have an American relative, Palo Santo
(*Bursera graveolens*). A denizen of dry tropical forests, it grows primar-
ily in Peru, Ecuador, and neighboring regions of South America but has
been found as far north as Arizona. Palo Santo is a sacred plant for
many indigenous American peoples (*palo santo* means "holy wood"),
but it is rapidly becoming endangered due to the loss of habitat and
overuse of its fragrant wood.

In the Fifth and Sixth Dynasties (between 2465 and 2323 BCE),
Egyptians imported Frankincense and Myrrh as offerings for the Gods,
for the process of mummification, for fumigation of homes, for medicine (for treating wounds and sores), and for personal hygiene. The resins were burned or added to oil, which was then applied to the body. A
bowl of what is thought to be Frankincense was even found in the tomb
of Tutankhamun.

In ancient Israel, according to the Torah, Myrrh and Frankincense
were used during Temple sacrifices.[45] Frankincense was also burned in
mosques and in Christian churches.

The LORD said to Moses, "Take the finest spices: of liquid myrrh 500 shekels, and of sweet-smelling cinnamon half as much, that is, 250, and 250 of aromatic cane, and 500 of cassia, according to the shekel of the sanctuary, and a hin of olive oil. And you shall make of these a sacred anointing oil blended as by the perfumer; it shall be a holy anointing oil. With it you shall anoint the tent of meeting and the ark of the testimony, and the table and all its utensils, and the lampstand and its utensils, and the altar of incense, and the altar of burnt offering with all its utensils and the basin and its stand. You shall consecrate them, that they may be most holy. Whatever touches them will become holy." . . .

The LORD said to Moses, "Take sweet spices, stacte, and onycha, and galbanum, sweet spices with pure frankincense (of each shall there be an equal part), and make an incense blended as by the perfumer, seasoned with salt, pure and holy. You shall beat some of it very small, and put part of it before the testimony in the tent of meeting where I shall meet with you. It shall be most holy for you." (Exodus 30)

Plutarch reported that the ancient Egyptians burned Frankincense at morning prayers in their temples, Myrrh at midday prayers, and *kyphi (kapet)*—an aromatic mixture made with mastic, Pine resin (or wood), Camel Grass, Mint, Sweet Flag, Cinnamon, Raisins, wine, and honey— in the evening. Certain Gods and Goddesses were associated with specific types of incense; for example, the Goddesses Hathor and Isis were strongly associated with Myrrh.

The newly converted Coptic Christians associated Mary with the Goddess Isis. The earliest images of Mary nursing the baby Jesus were based on older images of Isis suckling the infant Sun God Horus. (Horus is reborn each year on December 25. Coincidence?) Another fine example of Egyptian influence in the Mary and Jesus story is the "Madonna and Child" page from the medieval Irish Book of Kells, which was drawn in the Coptic (Egyptian) style. Is it possible that the three magi-astrologers who bestowed gifts of Frankincense and Myrrh were also honoring Jesus's mother, Mary?

Two thousand years ago, gold, Frankincense, and Myrrh were standard gifts to honor a king or deity in the Middle East. Gold was prized as an incorruptible precious metal, Frankincense as a costly and rare perfume or incense, and Myrrh as an incense and anointing oil. Ancient inscriptions tell us that Seleucus II Callinicus, king of the Seleucid empire from 246 to 225 BCE, offered all three to the God Apollo at the temple in Miletus in 243 BCE.[46]

Frankincense was also a valuable pain-relieving agent; it has an active ingredient that can help relieve arthritis and heal wounds. Perhaps the gift of Frankincense to the newborn Jesus was meant to affirm his role as a healer. Other symbolism can be found in the gold representing his kingship, Frankincense as a symbol of his role as a priestly rabbi, and Myrrh, which was used in embalming mixtures, as a prefiguration of his death.[47]

Production of the fragrant resins of Myrrh and Frankincense involves scoring the bark of the trees, collecting the exudate that seeps from the wounds, and drying it.

Medicinal Properties of Frankincense

Frankincense is anti-inflammatory, expectorant, antiseptic, anxiolytic (reduces anxiety), and antineurotic (counters neurosis). Its anti-inflammatory action has been shown useful in treating rheumatism, ulcerative colitis, irritable bowel syndrome, bronchitis, sinusitis, and asthmas. Its constituent boswellic acids have been shown to prevent tumors from spreading, especially cells of leukemia and glioblastoma.[48] Other uses are also being explored, including its benefit for Crohn's disease and osteoarthritis.

Dosing guidelines suggest that adults take 300 to 500 milligrams of Frankincense orally two or three times a day.

> **CAUTION:** The resin has not been rigorously studied, so pregnant and breastfeeding women should probably avoid using it medicinally. Frankincense can stimulate blood flow in the uterus and pelvis, accelerating menstrual flow and possibly inducing miscarriage. In some individuals it can cause nausea, acid reflux, diarrhea, and skin rashes. Do not take it in combination with other anti-inflammatory medications such as nonsteroidal anti-inflammatory drugs (NSAIDs).[49]

Frankincense Essential Oil

Frankincense essential oil (olibanum) is reported to ease stress, boost immune function, relieve pain, treat dry skin, reverse signs of aging, fight cancer, and improve heart rate, breathing, and blood pressure, among other things.[50]

Combine 1 or 2 drops of the essential oil with a carrier oil, such as Jojoba, Sweet Almond, or Avocado oil, and apply to the skin or add to the bath in small amounts. For an inhalation, sprinkle 1 or 2 drops of the essential oil onto a cloth or tissue and smell it, or use the oil in a diffuser or vaporizer.

Medicinal Properties of Myrrh

Myrrh can be used in gargles and mouthwashes to treat mouth sores and sore throat. It is used internally for chest complaints and coughs, bad breath, loose teeth, and weak gums. As a disinfectant, it is useful in wound washes and douches. Powdered Myrrh can be applied to clean wounds as a disinfectant dressing.

Infusion: Bring 2 cups of water to a boil and add 1 teaspoon of Myrrh. Allow the brew to steep for 3 to 5 minutes, covered, then strain. Take in teaspoon doses five or six times a day.

Gargle: Bring 2 cups of water to a boil and add 1 teaspoon of Myrrh and 1 teaspoon of boric acid. Cover, let steep for 30 minutes, then strain.

Tincture: Take 2 to 5 drops in water four times a day, not with meals.[51]

> **CAUTION: Don't overuse this herb internally. Amounts greater than 2 to 4 grams can cause kidney irritation and heart rate changes. It is usually safe when applied to the skin or diluted in a bath but can cause some side effects, such as rash.**

Myrrh Essential Oil

The essential oil has antimicrobial properties, especially when combined with Frankincense essential oil. It has been used for colds, coughs, insomnia, digestive discomfort, and sore throat. It reduces inflammation, stimulates the immune system, alleviates pain, and promotes wound healing.

It is believed to transmit messages to the limbic system, a brain region involved in controlling emotions, thus easing nervous conditions and calming the heart.[52]

Combine 1 or 2 drops of Myrrh essential oil with a carrier oil, such as Jojoba, Sweet Almond, or Avocado oil, and apply to the skin or add to the bath in small amounts. For an inhalation, sprinkle 1 or 2 drops of the oil onto a cloth or tissue and smell it, or use the essential oil in a diffuser or vaporizer.

Magical Uses

The scents of Frankincense and Myrrh bring deep healing on a mental, emotional, physical, and spiritual level. Use them as incense to heal anyone in emotional or physical pain. You can make a healing poppet out of blue cloth, stuffed with medicinal herbs and a "signature," such as a bit of hair from the person who needs healing, their picture, or even their name written on some parchment or Birch bark. Anoint the poppet with oils of Myrrh and Frankincense. Speak to the poppet, saying, "You are (person's name) and you are perfectly healed in mind, body, and spirit," while you visualize the person happy and well.

Use Frankincense and Myrrh to cleanse your home or ritual space and to attract abundance, love, and the highest spiritual energies. Put Frankincense in a yellow or gold sachet and carry it to attract good luck. Use the oils to anoint your ritual tools and the altar. Anoint your third eye, heart, and belly with the oils to amplify self-confidence, love, and compassion. Burn the resins or place them under your pillow for peaceful sleep and dreams.

Frankincense and Myrrh at Yuletide

Frankincense and Myrrh are suitable offerings for Sun Gods, such as Apollo, Bast, Belenos, Ra, Áine, or Grainne. Use them in Yule rituals to celebrate the return of the Sun. Burn Frankincense and Myrrh resins on charcoal or toss them into the ritual fire. The smoke will carry the scent to the Sky World of the deities.[53]

🌿 Spiritual Face Cream

Use Frankincense and Myrrh to craft a mystical, spiritual elixir that you can use to smooth wrinkles and attract high spiritual energies and psychic protection, any time you need it.

This recipe makes about ½ cup. The coconut oil must be solid to prepare the cream; if yours is liquid, refrigerate it until it solidifies. The beeswax is not required, but it will keep your face cream solid in the heat of summer. To melt it, use a double boiler or bain-marie.

Makes about ½ cup

> ½ cup organic solid coconut oil
>
> ¼ teaspoon vitamin E oil
>
> 5 drops frankincense essential oil
>
> 3 drops myrrh essential oil
>
> 1 tablespoon beeswax, melted (optional)

Whip the coconut oil with a hand mixer for 1 to 3 minutes, until it is light and fluffy.

Mix the vitamin E oil and essential oils into the whipped coconut oil. Add the melted beeswax, if you are using it, and continue to whip with a hand mixer until all the ingredients are thoroughly combined.

Spoon the cream into clean glass or plastic jars, cap, and store in a cool, dark place.

Adapted from Tiffany Marie's "Frankincense and Myrrh Beauty Face Cream," Coconut Mama (website), July 9, 2016.

Ginger
(*Zingiber officinale*)
·················· 🌿 ··················

And I had but one penny in the world, thou should'st have
it to buy gingerbread.

WILLIAM SHAKESPEARE,
LOVE'S LABOUR'S LOST (CA. 1595)

The word *ginger* comes from Sanskrit *sringavera* (root shaped like a horn). The compound *gingerbread* comes from the Old French *gingebras* (preserved ginger), which morphed into *gyngebreed* in Middle English and then into *gingerbread*.

Ginger was first cultivated in ancient China, where it was used as medicine, and eventually it spread to Europe via the Silk Road. In the Middle Ages, it was valued for its ability to preserve meat (and disguise the taste of meat past its prime). Henry VIII used a Ginger compound in an attempt to build his resistance to the plague, and Ginger is still used as a remedy for nausea, seasickness, and other stomach ailments.

The earliest known gingerbread recipe comes from Greece in 2400 BCE. The Chinese developed recipes in the tenth century, and European versions appeared by the late Middle Ages. Hard gingerbread cookies, sometimes gilded with gold leaf and shaped like kings, queens, and animals, became a staple treat at medieval fairs, where they were known as "fairings." The shapes of the cookies changed with the seasons; flower-shaped cookies appeared in spring and bird-shaped confections in the fall.

Gingerbread also held spiritual meaning in the Middle Ages. Monks made it to feed the hungry, but also to give religious instruction by pressing it into molds carved with images of saints or biblical scenes.

According to traditional lore, Queen Elizabeth I invented gingerbread men when she had them prepared as gifts for officials visiting her court. Gingerbread houses first appeared in Germany in the sixteenth century. Their popularity soared in the 1800s when the Brothers Grimm published the story of Hansel and Gretel, in which the main characters stumble upon a house made entirely of gingerbread, deep in the forest. Queen Victoria, who adored all things German, popularized gingerbread in England. Gingerbread came to North America with European colonists and was served by George Washington's mother, Mary Ball Washington, to the Marquis de Lafayette when he visited her home in Fredericksburg, Virginia.[54]

Medicinal Properties

Ginger is one of my favorite, go-to household remedies. I always keep a fresh root ready for use on the counter. In Chinese medicine, it's said to promote internal secretions. In other words, it gets things moving up and out of your system. For example, for people sick with bronchitis or flu, it warms the body and pushes out phlegm. It also improves blood circulation and reduces blood sugar levels and blood pressure. As an anti-inflammatory, it can be prepared as a tea to ease the pain of rheumatism and arthritis.

Ginger is a deep-acting digestive stimulant that eases nausea, stomach spasms, and vomiting. Ginger tea, prepared from the fresh (not dried) root, can help with morning sickness when taken in small amounts and can be used to relieve the nausea of chemotherapy. Ginger capsules can be taken to prevent seasickness. They help ease motion sickness, too, in both humans and animals.

Ginger is also an antiseptic and can be prepared as a wash for cuts and scratches.

Ginger is perhaps best known for its ability to ease the symptoms and aid the recovery of people suffering from colds, flu, and similar illnesses. For example:

For colds, bronchitis, sore throat, and fever: Simmer about 2 inches of the fresh root, sliced, per cup of water, covered, for 20 minutes. Take ¼ cup four or five times a day. Add honey and Lemon to taste.

For illness with chills or particularly dense and sticky phlegm: Prepare Ginger tea as described above, and add a pinch of Cinnamon. Or try Barley soup with grated Ginger added to it, or add strong Ginger tea to a hot bath.

For fever: Combine 1 teaspoon of grated fresh Ginger root, 1 teaspoon of grated fresh Horseradish, and 1 teaspoon of Soy sauce. Let marinate for 2 hours. Add to 1 cup of hot bancha tea and drink. Get into bed and bundle up.

To open the sinuses: Combine 8 ounces of V8 juice with freshly grated Ginger root, freshly grated Horseradish, Cayenne Pepper, two or three cloves of freshly chopped Garlic, and the juice of half a Lemon in a blender. Blend and drink.

CAUTION: Do not take Ginger in medicinal doses for 2 weeks before a scheduled surgery, as it can interfere with blood clotting. Do not use it with other agents that interfere with blood clotting, such as Garlic, Ginseng, Ginkgo, aspirin, heparin, or warfarin. Do not combine with other medicines for motion sickness. Do not take it in combination with medications to lower blood sugar, as Ginger can theoretically increase their effects and cause a steep drop in blood glucose levels.[55]

Magical Uses

An herb of Mars and the Sun, and of earth and fire, spicy-hot ginger speeds up and enhances all magical spells. It is used especially to create passion and to heat up love spells. The powder can be sprinkled into your wallet to increase money, or a root planted to attract wealth (bury a root from the supermarket in a flower pot, water it well, and place it in a sunny window).

Eat or drink ginger before performing magic of any kind to empower yourself for success. Put it in a Spirit bag and wear it to promote good health and protection. Use the tea as a wash for magical blades. Sprinkle powdered Ginger in the yard to avert trouble.

A root that looks like a human form is an especially powerful magical ally that protects against evil Spirits and bad dreams. Dry such a root for long-term use, keep it wrapped in a white cloth, and place it in a nicely decorated box. "Feed" the root with a sprinkle of spirits or Florida Water once in each Moon cycle, and bring it out as needed.[56]

Kitchen Witches and Hearth Druids might make gingerbread or ginger cookies in the tradition of the Elizabethan age, when lovers exchanged spicy gingerbread as a love token. Those who were searching for mates or hoping to ward off evil devoured heart-shaped pieces. Eating gingerbread rabbits was said to increase fertility, and Witches reportedly made gingerbread figures and ate them to cause the death of their enemies.[57]

Ginger at Yuletide

Make spicy gingerbread, gingerbread men, or a gingerbread house. Your magical intent will determine the shapes you create.

Gingerbread Cookies

Use cookie cutters or cut and shape your own, as Queen Elizabeth I once did. Note that the dough has to be chilled for at least 3 hours and up to 2 days. Rolled out thin, the cookies are crisp and cracker-like. Rolled out thick, they are moist and plump. These spicy treats will jump-start any magical endeavor.

Makes about 3 dozen 3-inch cookies

> 3 cups organic all-purpose flour, plus more for rolling out
>   the dough
> 1 teaspoon baking soda
> 1½ teaspoons ground cinnamon
> 1½ teaspoons ground ginger
> 1 teaspoon ground allspice
> 1 teaspoon ground cloves
> ½ teaspoon sea salt
> ½ teaspoon freshly ground black pepper
> 1–2 tablespoons freshly grated organic ginger, for extra
>   potency (optional)
> 8 tablespoons (1 stick) organic unsalted butter, at room
>   temperature
> ¼ cup vegetable shortening, at room temperature
> ½ cup packed organic light brown sugar
> ⅔ cup unsulfured molasses
> 1 free-range organic egg
> Royal icing, for decoration (optional; see recipe 177)

Sift the flour, baking soda, cinnamon, powdered ginger, allspice, cloves, salt, and pepper all together through a wire sieve into a medium bowl. Mix in the fresh ginger, if using, and set aside.

In a large bowl, beat the butter and vegetable shortening until well combined. Add the brown sugar and beat until the mixture is light in texture and color. Beat in the molasses and egg.

Adapted from Rick Rodgers's "Gingerbread Cookies 101," Foodnetwork.com (website) post from Rodgers's *Christmas 101* (Random House, 1999).

With a wooden spoon, gradually mix the flour mixture into the butter mixture to make a stiff dough.

Divide the dough into two thick disks and wrap each disk in plastic wrap. Refrigerate for at least 3 hours and up to 2 days.

When you're ready to make cookies, preheat the oven to 350°F. Set the oven racks in the top and bottom thirds of the oven.

Remove one disk of dough from the refrigerator, keeping the other disk refrigerated until you're ready to use it. Let stand at room temperature until the dough is just warm enough to roll out without cracking, at least 10 minutes.

Place the dough on a lightly floured surface and sprinkle its top with flour. Roll it out $1/8$ inch thick, being sure that the dough isn't sticking to your work surface (dust your work surface with more flour as needed). For softer cookies, roll out the dough slightly thicker.

Cut out cookie shapes and transfer them to nonstick baking sheets, placing the cookies 1 inch apart.

Gently knead the scraps together and form them into another disk. Wrap and chill for 5 minutes before rolling out again to cut out more cookies.

Bake the cookies two sheets at a time, switching the positions of the sheets from top to bottom and back to front halfway through baking, until the edges of the cookies are set and crisp, 10 to 12 minutes.

Let the cookies cool on the baking sheets for 2 minutes, then transfer them to wire racks to cool completely.

Decorate, if desired, with icing.

Note: I doubled the amount of spice from the original recipe, which some had reported as too bland. The cookies can be stored in airtight containers at room temperature for up to 1 week.

Royal Icing

Royal icing can made up to 2 days ahead of time, stored in an airtight container with a moist paper towel pressed directly on the icing surface, and refrigerated. You can substitute fresh egg whites for the powdered egg whites and water, but be sure your eggs are good (see page 159).

Practice your decorating skills on aluminum foil or waxed paper before you begin icing the cookies. Once applied, the icing will harden into shiny white lines.

1 pound (4½ cups) organic confectioners' (powdered) sugar

2 tablespoons dried egg-white powder

6 tablespoons water

In a medium bowl, beat the confectioners' sugar, egg-white powder, and water until combined. Beat faster, scraping down the sides of the bowl often, until the mixture is very stiff, shiny, and thick enough to pipe.

To pipe line decorations, you'll need a pastry bag fitted with a tube with a small writing tip about ⅛ inch wide. To fill the pastry bag, fold back the top of the bag to form a cuff. Hold the bag in one hand, or place it in a tall glass. Using a rubber spatula, scoop the icing into the bag. Then unfold the cuff and twist the top of the bag closed.

Squeeze the icing down to fill the tube. Test your icing on a piece of waxed paper or aluminum foil, and then you're ready to decorate.

Hawthorn
(*Crataegus monogyna, Crataegus laevigata*)

A member of the Rose family, Hawthorn is a traditionally ornamental plant that also has profound healing and magical properties. Ancient Irish bards used prickly Hawthorn in cursing magic. They pierced a poppet with the thorns while reciting a satire, every day for a month, with their back to a Hawthorn tree. Witches were said to use the large thorns as sewing needles to embroider a curse or a blessing onto cloth.

In Celtic traditions, Hawthorns were used as "rag trees." Petitioners would take a strip of cloth and dip it into a holy well, then touch the cloth to whichever part of them is ailing, and finally tie it to a Hawthorn tree that overhung the holy well. As the cloth rotted away, it was said, so would their disease.

According to Celtic lore, a solitary Hawthorn growing on a hill, especially if a water source sat nearby, was said to mark an entrance to the land of Fairy.[*]

Today, England's most famous Hawthorn is the Glastonbury

---

[*]For a detailed look at Hawthorn and other trees used by the Celts for healing, spirituality, and magic, please see my books *A Druid's Herbal of Sacred Tree Medicine* (Destiny Books, 2008) and *Tree Medicine Tree Magic* (Pendraig Publishing, 2017).

Thorn. According to legend, the uncle of Jesus, Joseph of Arimathea, came to Britain to purchase tin, possibly accompanied by the teenaged Jesus. Arriving at Glastonbury, Joseph climbed Wearyall Hill and drove his staff into the ground, whereupon it immediately burst into flower, growing into a Hawthorn tree that, unusually, flowered twice a year, in May and then again at Christmas.

Other accounts say that Joseph came to proclaim the Gospel and to hide the Grail cup (although why he would sail all the way to England just to hide the cup escapes me). Joseph then founded Glastonbury Abbey in Somerset, in southwest England. At least that's what the good monks said. They also claimed that King Arthur was buried there, which was very good for the pilgrimage trade.

The original Hawthorn is long gone, but many cuttings survived and its descendants now grow all around Glastonbury. In times past, the queen of England was traditionally sent a sprig of the winter-blooming hawthorn, which was presented to her for her Christmas table, usually by the mayor of Glastonbury, often accompanied by students. The only way to propagate this twice-blooming hawthorn variety is from cuttings, since it does not grow from seed.[58]

Medicinal Properties

Hawthorn's use as a heart medicine was reported by the Greek physician Dioscorides in the first century. Modern medical research confirms that Hawthorn is effective for strengthening heart contractions, increasing blood flow to the heart, lowering LDL cholesterol and triglyceride levels, and modulating blood pressure, and Hawthorn extract can decrease fatigue and shortness of breath in cases of congestive heart failure.

Hawthorn has so many specific benefits for the heart that I think of it as a general tonic for just about all heart conditions. The ripe red berries, gathered after the first frost, are tinctured for these conditions, as are the flowers and young leaves in the spring. The two types of tinctures can be combined to make a potent healing tonic for the heart.

Hawthorn berries are antioxidant rich, making them a valuable nutritive remedy for conditions such as some cancers and infections, type 2 diabetes, asthma, and premature skin aging. They also are anti-inflammatory, vasodilatory (expanding blood vessels, meaning they can help lower blood pressure), mildly sedative (useful in treating anxiety), and rich in fiber, aiding digestion and constipation.[59]

On a spiritual level, the flower essence aids a person in giving and receiving love, increasing courage, expressing love, and healing heartache.[60]

Both the young leaves and flowers and the ripe berries are edible. To take them as medicine:

Berry tea: Simmer 1 to 2 teaspoons per cup of water, covered, for 20 minutes. Take ¼ cup up to three times a day.

Tincture: Take 20 drops of tincture in water or herbal tea up to three times a day.

Berry powder: Add 1 to 2 teaspoons to smoothies, juice, or water.[61]

> **CAUTION: In some individuals, Hawthorn can cause dizziness, nausea, and digestive symptoms. Do not use it in combination with medications for heart failure, as negative interactions could occur (I have seen very dramatic drops in blood pressure in several people who used Hawthorn with other heart medications). There is no data available regarding Hawthorn for people who are pregnant and breastfeeding, so use it with caution.[62]**

Magical Uses

Hawthorn is an herb of Mars and of fire. The word *haw* means "hedge," and thorny Hawthorn bushes were once grown into stout hedges to protect property—the original barbed wire! The berry-rich hedges also provided food and shelter for birds and other wildlife as well as heart-protective medicine for their human gardeners. Think of Hawthorn as a stout defender who can protect you physically, psychically, and emotionally, and use it in magical work devoted to those outcomes.

Hawthorn at Yuletide

At Yuletide, you can work the bright red berries into wreaths, centerpieces, and other greenery. Each winter I fill the flower pots near my front door with twigs laden with red Hawthorn berries, as well as

Cedar (*Thuja occidentalis*) and Pine boughs, branches with red Sumac berries, and sprigs of Holly. This makes a cheery welcome for visitors that lasts until spring.

For decorating indoors, you can fill a shallow bowl with sand and insert red candles and branches of Hawthorn, with its red berries, to make a splendid centerpiece. Add sprigs of Rose hips and branches of Cedar, Holly, Laurel, or Pine if you have them.

You can also make a Hawthorn cordial and share it with your loved ones.

🍃 A Hawthorn Cordial for the Heart

You could take a dropperful or two of this daily for heart health, sip it straight as a cordial after dinner, or dilute it with sparkling water for a healthy low-alcohol treat. The rosy-colored elixir would make a splendid Yule gift!

Pick your hawthorn berries in the fall after the first frost, when they have turned red. (You can also pick the flowers and very young leaves in spring, cover them with brandy, and steep them all summer. Strain out the liquid for use with the berries in the fall. The leaves, flowers, and berries are all tonics for the heart.) Purchase dried berries from an herb store if you can't pick the berries yourself.

Makes about ½ gallon

> 4 cups freshly picked hawthorn berries (or 2 cups dried),
> whole or crushed
> 2 whole vanilla beans
> 2 cinnamon sticks
> 1 tablespoon cardamom pods
> ½ gallon brandy
> 1 cup raw, local honey (or more or less, to taste)

Place the berries and spices in a large jar. Pour the brandy into the jar. Let infuse for 4–6 weeks (or until the Winter Solstice), shaking the jar once a day. Strain the liqueur into another large jar. Stir in the honey. Decant the cordial into bottles.

Adapted from Mason Hutchison's "Homemade Hawthorn Berry Elixir for Heart Health," Mountain Rose Herbs (website), January 25, 2019.

Hibiscus
(*Hibiscus rosa-sinensis, Hibiscus sabdariffa*)
·················· ✻ ··················

In Chinese folklore, Hibiscus flowers are associated with wealth, personal power, and fame. Giving someone Hibiscus signifies admiration or a wish for good fortune. In Malaysia, the flower's five petals represent diverse ethnic groups living in harmony.

In Victorian England, Hibiscus was a symbol of womanhood and delicate feminine beauty. Presenting a woman with a Hibiscus flower was an acknowledgment of her loveliness.

Red Hibiscus flowers are associated with passion, romance, and love, while pink flowers symbolize platonic love and caring. The white flowers imply innocence and purity, and purple ones imply knowledge, wisdom, and mystery. Yellow flowers mean happiness, fortune, and good luck, and orange flowers symbolize health, healing, and vitality.[63]

In Japan, Hibiscus symbolizes gentleness and hospitality, while in South Korea, it alludes to the afterlife and immortality. In Hindu mythology, the red Hibiscus carries the meaning of primal energy. It is the flower of Kali and Ganesha and is a proper gift for these deities.

In Greek lore, Adonis transformed into a Hibiscus to distract Aphrodite and Persephone and stop them from fighting with each other. For the ancient Egyptians, Hibiscus was a flower of love and lust.

In the Caribbean, Hibiscus petals are often made into tea and shared as hospitality. In Hawaii, a woman will wear a Hibiscus flower behind her left ear to show she has a mate. Wearing it behind her right ear means she is available. Leis are made with Hibiscus flowers as a symbol of joy and welcome.

A Filipino legend tells the story of a man named Gumeng who fell in love with a Diwata (water nymph) named Mula. Love between a mortal and a Diwata was forbidden by the Gods, but the two lovers just couldn't stand to be apart. One day the Gods sent a Demon to kill Gumeng for his transgression. The Demon snuck up behind Gumeng and stabbed him in the back, and Gumeng fell to the ground bleeding.

When Mula discovered him, she was devasted. She tried to save him with her Fairy magic, to no avail. Brokenhearted, she took the dagger to her own heart and fell to the ground, bleeding to death next to her lover. As Gumeng and Mula died, the Earth opened and pulled them into her healing embrace, leaving no trace of them behind. Soon after, a sprout emerged from the ground in the exact spot where the lovers had fallen. That tiny sprout grew to become a beautiful Hibiscus bush.[64]

Spiritually, Hibiscus flowers symbolize the Divine Feminine, the ability to create and nurture life. Like the butterfly, the flowers are short-lived. The butterfly and the Hibiscus are both totems that relate to seizing the moment and catching joy as it flies. Bees, bats, and hummingbirds feed on hibiscus, making them related totems as well.

Medicinal Properties

Hibiscus has been used since ancient times as a curative agent. The Egyptians used Hibiscus tea as a refrigerant (to lower body temperature), to treat heart and nerve diseases, and as a diuretic. In Africa, the tea was taken for constipation, cancer, liver disease, and colds, and a poultice of the leaves was applied to wounds. In Iran, the tea is a common treatment for high blood pressure.

Hibiscus is loaded with antioxidants. Ongoing modern research is proving that Hibiscus can reduce blood pressure and cholesterol levels, help ease dry coughs, lower a fever, and possibly help prevent obesity and fatty buildup in the liver. It also has anticancer properties.

To prepare a tea, pour boiling water over the dried flowers (2 teaspoons of dried flowers per cup of hot water) and let steep, covered, for about 20 minutes. Drink a cup, hot or cold two or three times per day.[65] (Note: Some people find the flavor very sour.)

CAUTION: Hibiscus tea is generally considered safe. More research is needed to determine a safe dosage for pregnant or breastfeeding women, children, and people with liver or kidney disease, so use it with caution in these cases. There is some evidence that it can affect the way the body processes acetaminophen (Tylenol), but this effect is likely very minimal.[66]

Magical Uses

Use red Hibiscus flowers in love and passion spells. Burn dried red Hibiscus flowers as incense, sleep with the fresh red flowers next to your bed, or place them under your pillow in order to engender love and lust. Do the same with the purple ones to inspire prophetic dreams.

🍃 A Hibiscus Love Spell

> A small glass jar with a lid
> A small piece of rose quartz
> 2 red hibiscus flowers
> 1 teaspoon dried coriander seed
> 1 teaspoon ground cinnamon
> Rose essential oil (or rose geranium essential oil as a substitute)
> Rose petals, if you have them (or rose geranium flowers as a substitute)
> A small red candle
> A few teaspoons of honey
> Matches

Begin by grounding and centering. Take a few deep breaths.

Put the rose quartz in the jar. Place the hibiscus flowers on top. Sprinkle in the coriander seed, cinnamon, and a couple of drops of rose oil. Add some rose petals, too, if you have them on hand. Screw the lid on tightly.

Anoint the red candle with a few drops of rose oil. Roll the anointed candle in some ground cinnamon and then in the honey (and rose petals, if you have them).

Attach the candle to the top of the jar by melting the bottom of the candle and then holding it in place on the lid until it sticks.

Light the candle wick.

Close your eyes and visualize the passionate love you want to call in. Feel that it is already happening and then send the energy into your jar.

Open your eyes and gaze into the candle flame. Feel the light of the candle

Adapted from Amaria Pollux's "The Passionate Magickal Properties of Hibiscus," WiccaNow (website), accessed July 2, 2021.

and the power of the flowers attracting and empowering the passion you desire.

Allow the candle to burn itself down, undisturbed.

You could do a similar candle spell with different colors of flowers and stones and appropriate herbs and scents. For example, you might use purple Hibiscus with amethyst for wisdom, yellow Hibiscus with gold for joy, pink Hibiscus with rose quartz for familial love, white Hibiscus with clear quartz for purification, and so on.

Hibiscus at Yuletide

Place some red Hibiscus flowers on the altar in honor of Kali and Ganesh. Ask Kali to remove all unpleasant obstacles left over from last year, and ask Ganesh to bring in prosperity and good luck for the new year. Serve a red Hibiscus libation at your Winter Solstice gathering, such as a tea or cordial, sangria (see the recipe below), or Jamaican sorrel (see page 122).

🌱 Hibiscus Sangria

Kitchen Witches and Hearth Druids will likely make use of this hibiscus-powered drink to engender love and passion. Apples and strawberries are fruits of love, the oranges and lemon bring in the energy of the returning Sun, the honey bestows sweetness, and the spices kindle just a touch of lust. What's not to like?

Makes 16 servings

> 6 cups water
> ¾ cup dried hibiscus petals
> ½ cup raw, local honey (or to taste)
> 2 cinnamon sticks
> 1 teaspoon ground cardamom
> 2 (750-milliliter) bottles rosé wine
> ¾ cup brandy
> ½ cup organic brown sugar
> ½ cup elderflower syrup (optional)

Adapted from chikalin's "Hibiscus Sangria," Allrecipes (website), accessed July 3, 2021.

¼ cup triple sec (or any clear, dry, orange-flavored liqueur,
such as Cointreau)

½ fresh organic pineapple, peeled, cored, and cut into
chunks

2 organic Granny Smith apples, cut into chunks

1 pint organic strawberries, cut into chunks

2 organic oranges, sliced and cut into small chunks

1 organic lemon, sliced and cut into small chunks

Sparkling water, if desired

Bring the water, hibiscus petals, honey, cinnamon sticks, and cardamom to
a simmer in a large pot. Remove from the heat and let steep, covered, for
1 hour, then strain.

Stir the wine, brandy, brown sugar, elderflower syrup, and triple sec into
the hibiscus water. Keep stirring until the sugar is dissolved. Then add the
pineapple, apples, strawberries, oranges, and lemon.

Refrigerate, covered, for at least 8 hours or overnight.

Serve as is, spooning some of the fruit into each glass. For a less alcoholic
drink, add a splash of sparkling water to each serving.

Holly
(*Ilex* spp.)

........................🌿........................

Heigh ho! sing heigh ho! unto the green holly:
Most friendship is feigning, most loving mere folly:
Then, heigh ho, the holly!
This life is most jolly."
WILLIAM SHAKESPEARE, *As You Like It* (CA. 1599)

Why do we decorate with Holly at Yuletide? The tradition goes back to
the days of the ancient Roman Saturnalia (December 17 through 23),
a festival dedicated to Saturn, the God of agriculture and husbandry,
when Romans would tie a bright sprig of Holly to the gifts they
exchanged.

In Norse tradition, Holly was sacred to Thor, God of thunder and
lightning, war, and fertility, and Holly plants were grown by the home

to prevent lightning strikes. Among the Gauls, Holly was sacred to Taranis, God of thunder and storms.

For the Pagan Celts, Holly was a warrior Spirit and a plant of protection, likely because prickly Holly leaves are fierce to the touch and the red berries resemble blood. The spikes on Holly leaves were said to ensnare any evil Spirits that might seek to enter at the dark of the year, so Holly was hung on entrances as a protective spell. It was also hung in the home to protect it from ill-intentioned Faeries, even as it gave kindlier Spirits a place to shelter from the chaos and cold of the season. Holly was once a favored winter food for deer and farm animals, and was planted near trees such as Oak to keep animals from disturbing the valuable timber.

In British Pagan tradition, the Holly tree symbolizes the waning of the Sun, commencing with the Summer Solstice, and the Oak tree symbolizes the waxing of the Sun, commencing with the Winter Solstice. This symbolism can be seen in the legend in which the Holly King battles the Oak King for dominance at the Solstices. The Oak King wins as the light half of the year comes in, while the Holly King dominates as the dark half of the year starts.

> *But the hue of his every feature*
> *Stunned them: as could be seen,*
> *Not only was this creature*
> *Colossal, he was bright green*
> *No spear to thrust, no shield against the shock of battle,*
> *But in one hand a solitary branch of holly*
> *That shows greenest when all the groves are leafless*
>
> SIR GAWAIN AND THE
> GREEN KNIGHT (CA 1370–1390)

A British seasonal ritual once involved both Holly and Ivy. A boy dressed in a suit of Holly leaves and a girl dressed in Ivy paraded around the village, carrying the energies of green nature through the town. They wore the evergreens as a way of guaranteeing that fertility would endure, even through the coldest and darkest days of winter.

In Scotland, from the Isle of Mull to Ross-shire, the McLean clan adopted Holly as its clan badge, worn by warriors in their caps when they went to battle.[67]

The Pre-Columbian indigenous North Americans of Cahokia, a large settlement near present day Saint Louis (800–1100 CE), and other First Nations peoples used Yaupon Holly (*Ilex vomitoria*) as a ceremonial drink. It was an herb of fertility, purification and life-renewal.[68]

When any culture lists a plant as "sacred" or "protective" and weaves stories around it, it is wise to pay attention, because that respect means the plant has profound practical value. Holly was once a medicine for fevers, coughs, and colds. It was a valuable winter fodder for the farm animals, and its wood was used to make charcoal, tool handles, and whips for plowmen and horse-drawn coaches.

Medicinal Properties

Holly leaves are loaded with antioxidants, making them a boost to the immune system.

Ilex aquifolium is the traditional English Holly (aka the common Holly, European Holly, or Mountain Holly) that we think of at Christmas. The leaves (not the berries, which are poisonous!) have been used by herbalists for centuries for gout, urinary issues, chronic bronchitis, rheumatism and arthritis (joint pain), fevers, and swelling and water retention. To prepare it as a tea, steep 2 teaspoons of dried leaves per cup of water, covered, for 20 minutes. Take ¼ cup four times a day, not with meals.

The leaves of *Ilex opaca,* White Holly also known as both American Holly and Winterberry, are used to cleanse the bowels, stimulate the heart, and increase urine flow. This makes another good noncaffeinated tea. Dry and crumble the leaves before use and steep 2 teaspoons of dried leaves per cup of water, covered, for 20 minutes.

A tea of *Ilex vomitoria,* Yaupon Holly, is a stimulant if not made too strong and an emetic if taken in very strong doses. Yaupon Holly young leaves have a very high caffeine content. Dry the leaves, then powder or crumble them (using a mortar and pestle). Bring water to a boil, take it off the stove, and pour it over the leaves. Allow the leaves to steep for about 5 minutes, using 1 teaspoon of leaves per cup of hot water. The same leaves can be used once or twice more, just steep them a few minutes longer.

The bark of *Ilex aurus llate,* Winterberry, makes a wash for skin eruptions and irritations. A tea of the root is good for fever and digestive upsets; to prepare it, simmer 1 teaspoon of root per cup of water, covered, for 20 minutes. Take 1 to 2 cups per day, cold.[69]

The leaves and twigs of *Ilex paraguariensis,* Yerba Maté, a common caffeinated drink in South America, can be prepared as a tea that is just as stimulating as coffee. It can benefit headaches, migraines, and fatigue and boost mental energy. Coffee addicts can use it to break themselves of the coffee habit.[70] Steep 1 tablespoon of the leaves in 8 ounces of water overnight, or brew with hot water as you would any tea. Add honey and Pineapple, Orange, or Lemon juice, as desired.[71] A tea made from the leaves (and those of *Ilex theezans*) is also blood-cleansing and diuretic.

CAUTION: The berries are poisonous and could be deadly, so keep them away from children. For some people, the leaf tea can cause diarrhea, nausea, vomiting, and stomach or intestinal issues. When swallowed, Holly leaf spines could puncture the inside of the mouth and other parts of the digestive tract. Due to the caffeine level and powerful active ingredients in Yaupon Holly and Yerba Maté teas, they are not recommended for pregnant or breastfeeding women. And data in general is lacking on the safety of Holly during pregnancy and breastfeeding, so it's best to avoid medicinal uses of Holly under those conditions.

Magical Uses

Hang Holly in the home for protection against lightning, poisoning, ill-intentioned Spirits, and sorcery. Holly is said to carry a male warrior spirit that is especially empowering for men, while Ivy embodies the feminine energies and is especially empowering for women. Use them together as Yuletide decorations.

Toss a sprig of Holly at a wild animal when you feel threatened, to make them lie down and leave you alone. Sprinkle an infusion of Holly water on a newborn baby to protect it. Use a wand of Holly wood to banish unwanted entities and Spirits.

For dream manifestation, pick nine Holly leaves and tie them in a white cloth. Seal the cloth with nine knots, blowing your intent into each knot after it is tied. Place the cloth under your pillow and allow it to enhance your dreams.

Holly is an herb of Mars. Feel its protective forces surrounding you as you sip a cup of the brew! Incidentally, the best Holly for decaffeinated tea is Gallberry or Inkberry (*Ilex glabra*), which tastes like orange pekoe without the caffeine. Dry and crumble the leaves before use and steep for about 5 minutes using 1 teaspoon per cup of freshly boiled water. See the Medicinal Properties above for other brews.

Reminder: *Never* **eat Holly berries of any species. They are poisonous!**

Holly at Yuletide

Hang boughs of Holly on the door and in the house at Yuletide and then burn the Holly decorations at Imbolc, leaving a sprig hanging somewhere in the house for luck and protection.

Enact a ritual battle between the Holly King and the Oak King. The Oak King wins in the end, of course, and ushers in the new season of Light.

Consider incorporating a ceremonial drink of Yaupon Holly into a Solstice rite in honor of the indigenous ancestors of this land (the Americas).

Make a Holly garland to drape over your Yule tree, fireplace, door, bannisters, or altar.

🍃 Make a Holly Garland

Clippers
Paddle (florist) wire, 22 gauge
Gloves (because Holly has sharp leaves)
Twine

Cut bunches of Holly with berries, about 6–8 inches in length. Consider adding in bunches of other evergreens such as Boxwood, Pine (and Pine cones), Cedar, Spruce, etc. Find these evergreens in nature or buy them at a garden center.

If you use Pine cones, wind a 10-inch length of wire around the bottom of each cone to make a "stem." Then you can attach the pine cones at random as desired.

Lay out a length of twine corresponding to how long you want your Holly garland to be. Along it, lay your Holly cuttings so they all face the same direction, 5 or 6 sprigs of Holly per bunch.

Wind the first bunch of 5 or 6 sprigs together with the floral wire (do not cut the wire, just keep using it continuously to wind and bind as you go down the length of string). Bind the first bunch to the top of your length of twine using the wire.

Make a second bunch of Holly or other evergreens, lay it over the stems of the first bunch, and bind it with wire. Keep going down the entire length of twine, binding the bottom of each bunch of greenery as you go.

When you reach the end of your length of twine, bind in one last bundle facing the opposite direction. Cut the wire and wrap the end around a bundle. If you notice any gaps just fill in with smaller bundles of greenery or pine cones as needed.

Hyssop
(*Hyssopus officinalis*)
·················· 🌿 ··················

Purge me with hyssop, and I shall be clean;
wash me, and I shall be whiter than snow.

PSALM 51:7

Native to southern Europe and Eurasia, Hyssop was considered an herb of purification in ancient Egypt and was used by priests, who ate it with their bread.[72] The Romans used it to make an herbal wine. In the Middle Ages, monks used it in their cooking. The peppery, bitter flavor was a seasoning for soups and sauces, disguised the taste of spoiled meats, and was believed to aid in the digestion of fats. It was considered a purifying tea and a medicine.

Tudor and Elizabethan knot gardens often included Hyssop, which was grown for strewing on floors, and early European colonists brought it with them to North America. It is listed among the seeds of John Winthrop Jr., who came to the American colonies in 1631.[73]

Today, Hyssop is still used as a flavoring for liqueurs such as absinthe, Chartreuse, and Bénédictine liqueur.

Medicinal Properties

Hyssop has traditionally been used for digestive issues, liver problems, gallbladder disease, gas, stomachaches, intestinal pain, and colic. It has an affinity for the upper respiratory tract and loosens mucus congestion; coughs, sore throats, colds, asthma, and flu all fall within its sphere of influence. For bronchitis and asthma, it can be mixed with Horehound (*Marrubium vulgare*). Combine it with Sage (*Salvia officinalis*) to make a gargle for sore throat.

It is also used to treat edema, urinary tract infections, poor circulation, and menstrual cramps, and, in a bath, to promote sweating. It is used topically as a wash or poultice for burns, bruises, wounds, infections, cold sores, genital herpes, and frostbite.[74]

Modern studies are confirming the uses ascribed to this plant by traditional herbalists for millennia. A 2014 study found that herbs in the Lamiaceae family, including Hyssop, may be able to destroy cancer cells, including breast cancers.[75] Another study determined that hyssop may be effective against ulcers in the digestive tract. A 2017 study showed that hyssop may indeed benefit asthma.[76] Other studies show that hyssop has antiaging properties for the skin and are confirming its antiviral properties.[77]

Specific applications include the following:

For a simple cold remedy: Steep 1 tablespoon of dried Hyssop flowers and leaves, or 3 tablespoons fresh, in 1 cup of freshly boiled water, covered, for 10 minutes. Strain, then stir in 1 tablespoon of honey and 1 teaspoon of Lemon juice and drink hot.

To make an infusion for other conditions: Steep 1 tablespoon of dried Hyssop per cup of freshly boiled water, covered, for 20 minutes. Take up to 1½ cups a day in tablespoon doses. Sweeten with honey for coughs and chest conditions.

To make a poultice: Pour freshly boiled water over the dried herb and let it sit until the plant matter is soft (about 15 minutes). Then spread the softened herb over a cloth and apply to the affected area.[78]

> CAUTION: Do not use Hyssop continuously for long periods of time. Hyssop leaves, flowers, and shoots are safe in small quantities (such as might be needed when consuming them for food) and for the duration of an acute illness. Children should not be given Hyssop as an herbal remedy. The essential oil may cause seizures in children and in some adults; avoid Hyssop if you have a history of epilepsy or seizures. Overuse of this herb or very high doses may also cause seizures. Hyssop can cause uterine contractions, so those who are pregnant should avoid it. Its effects can be passed to an infant through breast milk, so those who are breastfeeding should also avoid it.[79]

Magical Uses

Hyssop is an herb of fire and of Jupiter; it is mainly an herb of protection and purification. On a psychic level, it has very high spiritual energies and can help you sort through difficulties and organize your life.

Hyssop repels evil forces, curses, and negative energies. Use branches of Hyssop to asperge people and sacred spaces. Burn the herb to cleanse and purify the home or the ritual area. Make a tea and use it to wash floors, windows, and doors of the home for purification and protection. Add Hyssop to a ritual bath for breaking hexes and curses, and carry it or wear the scent for protection from negative energies.

Kitchen Witches and Hearth Druids can incorporate Hyssop's protective energies into both main courses and desserts. It has a strong aromatic flavor resembling a cross between Mint and Sage. Sprinkle the fresh flowers on salads or desserts as a decorative garnish. Use the leaves and young shoots in soups, sauces, and casseroles.

According to traditional lore, Hyssop has an affinity with dragons. Use it to enhance communication with them.[80]

Hyssop at Yuletide

Hang bunches of Hyssop in the home as protection from mischievous Spirits that roam the Earth at the darkest time of year. Burn the herb or use it as a wash on floors and entrances to ensure peace and block negativity at family gatherings.

🍃 Four Thieves Vinegar

According to legend, this mixture was used in France during the scourge of the Black Death. Thieves would cover their bodies and masks with the vinegar as they stole out on moonless nights to steal from the houses of the dead. According to reports, it did keep them safe from illness; the herbs and vinegar actually have strong antibacterial and antiviral properties.

This is just one version; different versions call for angelica, camphor, cloves, horehound, elecampane, juniper, marjoram, meadowsweet, wormwood, and other herbs. Mix and match the herbs as you see fit, or according to their magical properties. Ideally, all the herbs you use will be fresh, but in the dark season of Yule you can make do with dried herbs; just halve the amounts you use.

You can pour this versatile vinegar across a doorway to stop evil from entering, use it to clean and disinfect kitchen surfaces, use it as a skin wash and healing agent, or simply pour it onto salads, braised meats, and vegetable dishes.

Makes about four cups.

2 tablespoons fresh anise hyssop

2 tablespoons fresh lavender flowers

2 tablespoons fresh marjoram

2 tablespoons fresh mint

2 tablespoons fresh rosemary

2 tablespoons fresh sage

4 cloves organic garlic, peeled and crushed

4 cups organic white wine vinegar

Adapted from Jenny McGruther's "Four Thieves Vinegar," Nourished Kitchen (website), July 19, 2011.

Place the herbs and garlic in a Mason jar. Cover the herbs with the vinegar and cap the jar (plastic caps are ideal because vinegar corrodes metal). Set in a sunny window and let steep—7 to 10 days for culinary use, or 6 months for a stronger curse-blocking potion.

Strain the liquid into another clean glass jar. Cap with a plastic lid; if you have only a metal lid, place a bit of waxed paper under it to prevent corrosion.

Store at room temperature.

Ivy
(Hedera helix)

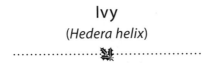

At Christmas tide Holly (the "holy tree"), Rosemary, Laurel, Bay, Arbor Vitae, and Ivy are hung up in churches, and are suitable also for the decoration of houses, with the important addition of Mistletoe (which, on account of its Druidic connection, is interdicted in places of worship). Ivy should only be placed in outer passages or doorways.

RICHARD FOLKARD, *PLANT LORE,*
LEGENDS, AND LYRICS (1884)

According to Greek mythology, as an infant the God Bacchus was originally named Kissos. His mother, Semele, abandoned him under an Ivy bush, and that's how Ivy (Kissos in Greek) got its name. A different account says that Kissos was the son of Bacchus, who danced for his father and suddenly dropped dead. The Goddess Gaea took pity on him and transformed him into an Ivy plant.

Ivy is sacred to Bacchus, and he wears a crown of it, intertwined with Grapevines. His thyrsus (a staff or spear tipped with an ornament, such as a Pine cone, that is carried by Bacchus and his followers) has Ivy on its top. At Bacchanalian festivals, worshippers wore Ivy crowns or chaplets of Ivy and Violets, and women in the processions carried Ivy garlands. It's said that the Bacchae—female followers of Bacchus— would drink a mixture of fermented Ivy, Fly Agaric, and Pine sap and then rampage around the countryside, tearing animals and humans to pieces.[81]

Ivy is also sacred to Dionysus, the Roman God of wine. In one story, Dionysus punished a ship of pirates for their lack of reverence toward him by filling their boat with Ivy and magically turning their oars into serpents. As a result, the pirates lost their minds and drowned themselves in the ocean.

At Greek weddings, the altar of Hymen was decorated with Ivy, and lengths of Ivy were presented to the couple as a symbol of the wedding knot. In Norse lore, Ivy was dedicated to Thor, the God of thunder, and offered to the Elf who was his messenger. In ancient Egypt, Ivy was dedicated to Osiris, a God who represented death and immortality.

At Medieval fairs, booths were once decorated with Ivy to show that wine was available for purchase within. Oddly, wearing a crown of Ivy was believed to allay drunkenness! In Germany, when cattle were first driven out to pasture, they were each given a crown of Ivy to wear as protection. It was also said that a person wearing an Ivy crown would be able to identify Witches.

It was an English custom to bind the last sheaf of the harvest with Ivy. The bundle, called the Harvest Bride or Maid of the Ivy, was said to bring bad luck to the farmer who harvested late.[82] Farmers believed in Ivy's apparently magical healing properties for grazing livestock, especially cattle, and fed garlands of Ivy to sick animals, who sometimes made a startling recovery. On some Shropshire farms in England, Ivy would be fed to every animal before midday on Christmas morning to ward off the Devil for a year.[83] In Ireland, Ivy provided winter fodder for the animals of poor families. A small wreath of protective herbs, bound with Ivy, might be placed under a churn to keep Witches and Faeries from stealing the milk.

Ivy, in combination with Holly, was a popular Christmas decoration in the Middle Ages. Ivy was thought to embody a clinging female nature, while Holly spoke of masculine, warrior-like qualities. But in some areas, it was believed that Ivy should never be brought into the house. As an old English rhyme states:

> *Nay my nay, hyt shall not be I wis,*
> *Let Holly have the maystry, as the maner ys.*
> *Holly stoud in the hall, fayre to behold,*

Ivy stoud without the dore, she ys ful sore a-cold.
Nay my nay.[84]

Maybe Ivy was feared due to its Bacchanalian and Dionysian connections. Or perhaps it was banished from the house simply because it was regarded as a female plant that needed to be controlled. That's pretty sexist, don't you think?

Medicinal Properties

Traditional herbalists use Ivy as a wash for burns, sores, cuts, and other skin problems, as well as for dandruff.

Ivy is anti-inflammatory, antiarthritic, antioxidant, antiviral, antispasmodic, antimicrobial, and antitumor. It can help remove toxins from the body and strengthens the blood vessels. It also relaxes the airway muscles, relieves coughing, and helps loosen phlegm, helping individuals who are suffering from allergies, asthma, bronchitis, and COPD.[85]

One study found that Ivy improves lung function in children with chronic bronchial asthma.[86] Another study showed that it helps with arthritis, inflammation, and even cancer.[87]

To prepare Ivy for medicinal use, steep about one handful of fresh leaves or a ¼ cup of dried leaves per cup of water for 20 minutes. Take ¼ cup or less of the tea, four times a day, for the duration of an acute illness (no longer). Small doses are said to dilate the blood vessels and large doses to constrict them.[88]

CAUTION: Use only the leaves, in small doses, for a short time. The berries are poisonous. In some people, large amounts of Ivy can cause nausea and vomiting. High doses may also break down red corpuscles by releasing their hemoglobin. Do not overuse this herb. A few individuals have experienced shortness of breath, swelling, reddening of skin, and itching, but this is rare. People who are pregnant or breastfeeding should avoid this plant. Children's cough syrup (Prospan, Panoto-S, Athos, Abrilar) or herbal drops (Prospan) containing Ivy leaf extract, taken three times a day, may be safe for up to 20 days.[89]

Magical Uses

Ivy is a feminine herb that can be carried or worn by women for luck and fertility. Woven into a bride's bouquet or crown, it symbolizes fidelity. A house covered with Ivy vines repels negative energies and averts accidents; you can hang an Ivy plant by your door to keep away unwanted guests and in a sick person's room to cheer them and promote healing.[90]

Ivy blooms in the fall, providing a final burst of pollen for the bees, and is a healing fodder for cattle. It is an herb of protection, healing, generosity, and abundance. Use Ivy in charms for fidelity and love. Bind a magical wreath of protection with strands of Ivy and hang it in the entranceway.

Ivy at Yuletide

Decorate your home with Ivy as you prepare for your Yuletide festivities. Invite the Gods Bacchus and Dionysus to bless a cheerful gathering (and make sure there is plenty of red wine on hand!). Twine some Ivy and Holly to decorate a God and Goddess altar.

🍃 Ivy Laundry Detergent

Ivy is far too toxic to use as a food or a beverage, so instead I am sharing this recipe for a homemade, organic laundry detergent. Ivy is loaded with natural saponins (bitter-tasting, usually toxic plant-derived compounds that foam in water). Think of it as imbuing your clothes with energies of abundance and protection. This would be a great project for someone who is already working to remove ivy from the walls of their house.

Makes enough for about 3½ loads of laundry

> Rubber kitchen gloves (because ivy irritates
> the skin)
> 60 ivy leaves
> A large pan or pot
> 4½ cups water

Adapted from Christelle Siohan and Cristina Rojas's "English Ivy Laundry Detergent," Permacrafters (website), accessed July 29, 2021.

A tea strainer or cheesecloth

Vinegar (optional)

Wearing rubber kitchen gloves, rinse the ivy leaves and then scrunch them up with your hands.

Place the leaves in the pan and add the water. Bring to a boil and let boil for 15 minutes, stirring every once in a while. Then simmer lightly for about a half hour in a pot with a lid.

Put on those rubber gloves again. Squeeze and scrunch the leaves by hand in the water, expressing their juice. Then fish out the leaves, giving them one last good squeeze, and discard them in your compost pile.

When the tea has cooled, filter it into a large glass jar using a tea strainer or cheesecloth. Store in the refrigerator for a few days; if you want to keep it at room temperature, add a little bit of vinegar to it (at a 1:5 ratio) as a preservative. (By the way, vinegar in the wash sweetens the load, removing the odors of mold and mildew.)

Use ¾ cup of ivy tea per load of wash. Don't use this detergent on heavily soiled clothing. It is perfect for woolens and delicate items.

Juniper
(*Juniperus* spp.)
·················· 🌿 ··················

Disce et odoratam stabulis accendere Cedrum.
But learn to burn within your sheltering rooms
 Sweet Juniper.
      VIRGIL, *GEORGIKA* (CA. 29 BCE)

Juniper is sacred to the Erinyes (the Furies), the Greek Goddesses of vengeance who attack anyone who violates an oath or swears falsely. The Greeks burned Juniper roots as incense to please the Underworld deities and burned the berries at funerals to ward off evil. For the Canaanites, Juniper was a symbol of the fertility Goddess Ashera or Astarte. The ancient Romans also burned it as incense on their altars, while in Norway and Sweden, floors were strewed with the tops of Juniper, which diffused a pleasant fragrance to the rooms. Queen Elizabeth I of England was said to favor Juniper as a strewing herb to fragrance her floors.

Juniper is an herb of protection; a hare will reputedly seek it out as a last refuge when being chased by hounds, and the scent of juniper is said to defeat the dog's sense of smell. Lore has it that the Virgin Mary and the infant Jesus once hid in a Juniper tree while being pursued and were sheltered and protected by the tree. In some parts of Italy, branches of Juniper are hung in stables and cattle sheds on Christmas Day to commemorate that event; they're also used to brush openings and cracks in house walls to prevent evil Spirits and disease from entering. In Bologna, it was once customary to distribute branches of Juniper to houses on Christmas Eve.

In Germany, you might once have called upon Frau Wachholder, the Spirit of Juniper, when you wanted thieves to relinquish their spoils. To invoke her, you would stand under a Juniper tree, bend a branch down to the ground, and hold it in place with a stone. You would then intone the name of the thief and demand that they return what they stole. When the goods were returned, you would go back to the tree to release the branch.[91]

Juniper was also once hung in and around houses, beehives, and stables to block spells and repel Witchcraft. Hung on a door, it was said to stop Witches, who would compulsively count the leaves, an impossible task, thus distracting them from their mischief making and driving them away for fear of being recognized.

In Scotland, the *saining* (purification) of the house ritual takes place at Hogmanay (New Year's Eve). First the house and livestock are blessed by water from a local stream or holy well. Then the woman of the house goes from room to room with a smoldering Juniper branch, filling the house with purifying smoke, or she may clean the hearth and then burn Juniper in it. Ideally, there is enough smoke to fumigate the contents of the house and the inhabitants thoroughly, after which everyone is revived with a wee dram of whiskey.[92]

The scent of burning Juniper is said to strengthen powers of clairvoyance and to empower contact with the Otherworld of the Gods, Spirits, and ancestors. From Pakistan to Siberia, shamans burn juniper and inhale its smoke to facilitate trance work.

Indigenous American peoples valued Juniper for its protective powers. Northwestern tribes used it to guard against ill-intentioned Witchcraft and to banish evil Spirits. The Dakota, Cheyenne, and Pawnee burned it for protection during storms. The Pueblo held that Juniper counteracts "ghost sickness," protecting those who handled the bodies of the dead and those who were grieving. Many Native American peoples used Juniper in medicine bundles and protective amulets.[93]

A solar herb, Juniper features in dream interpretations. It is considered unlucky to dream of the tree itself, especially if the dreamer is ill. To dream of gathering the berries in winter denotes prosperity. To dream of the berries themselves signifies that the dreamer will soon achieve great honor or the birth of a male child.[94]

Juniper berries have long been used in the production of gin, giving the spirit its distinctive flavor. In medieval times they were also used in Scotland to flavor whiskey. The crushed berries are a traditional seasoning for meat dishes, especially wild game and fatty meats, as well as desserts and even Lemon sherbet. Juniper wood is sometimes added to the coals over which meat is being cooked to enhance its flavor.

Medicinal Properties

The earliest recorded medicinal use of Juniper comes from an Egyptian papyrus dating to 1500 BCE that contains a recipe using the berries to cure tapeworm infestations. The Romans used the berries for purification and for stomach ailments.[95] Modern herbalists use the berries whole or in tea to strengthen digestion and for all kinds of gastrointestinal infections and cramps.

This is another herb that should not be overused or taken for a long period of time, as it can irritate the kidneys and urinary tract. However, it is taken for kidney and bladder issues and is a helpful diuretic for cardiac and kidney edema.

Juniper essential oil can be used in a vaporizer to help with lung infections and coughs.

To prepare Juniper as a tea, steep 1 teaspoon of crushed berries per ½ cup of hot water for 10 minutes, covered, then strain. Take up to 1 cup a day in ¼-cup doses. You can also chew a few berries (no more than three) daily.[96]

> **CAUTION: Do not use Juniper if you are pregnant or breastfeeding, as it can cause miscarriage and its effect on breastfeeding infants is unknown. Diabetics should avoid it, too, as it can drastically lower blood sugar. It can irritate the stomach and intestinal tract of some individuals (try a small amount and see how it affects you before extended use). It can make blood pressure harder to control. Stop taking it 2 weeks before a scheduled surgery.[97]**

Magical Uses

Juniper is an herb of fire and sacred to Apollo and to Ashera/Astarte. Use it as a ritual offering or incense to honor these and other Gods and Goddesses, and as an herb of protection any time your home or animals are threatened with bad luck or disease. Burn Juniper when doing divination or seeking clairvoyance.

Use Juniper oil, branches, or berries in antitheft and protection spells. Carry the berries on your person and place them in your car to block thieves, and make an offering to Frau Wachholder as you do this. Grow Juniper near your door to protect your house.

Use the berries in love spells to attract men, and add a tea or vinegar tincture of the berries to your bathwater for the same purpose. Steep the berries in drinks to increase male potency.[98]

Juniper at Yuletide

Burn Juniper in your house, barn, and ritual area at Solstice to purify these spaces and welcome in the new Sun cycle. Burn Juniper as incense on the altar in honor of Apollo, the Sun God. Hang Juniper boughs on gateposts and doors to repel troublesome Spirits and to preserve good energies in the home during the Yuletide season.

⟡ Homemade Lox: A Scandinavian-Style Appetizer for Your Yule Feast

Hearth Druids will appreciate this recipe, which features the sacred Salmon of Wisdom, cured with purifying salt, juniper berries, and rosemary. Dill is an herb of protection from evil forces, the lemons carry solar energies, and black pepper opens the "third eye," the ability to see beyond the physical world.

Lay the fish slices on lightly toasted whole-grain bread to carry the luck of the harvest from the old year to the new. Slather on a bit of organic yellow butter on the toasted bread as homage to the returning Sun. Garnish with a whole sprig or sprinkling of dill.

Note: *Farm-raised salmon have a poor diet (fish pellets) and less omega-3 fatty acids, which are known to lower the risk of heart disease. Always choose wild-caught salmon if you can find it.*

Makes about 12 servings

> 1 (2-pound) filet king salmon, center (thick) cut
> 12 whole juniper berries
> 1 teaspoon whole peppercorns
> ½ cup kosher salt (or smoked salt and smoked paprika for a smoky flavor)
> ⅛ cup organic sugar
> Zest from 2 large organic lemons
> ¼ cup chopped rosemary
> ¼ cup vodka
> Fresh or dried dill, for garnish

Line a sheet pan with plastic wrap. Place the salmon skin side down on the sheet pan and pat dry.

Crush the juniper berries and peppercorns in a mortar and pestle or grind them coarsely, then transfer them to a small bowl. Add the salt, sugar, lemon zest, and rosemary and mix thoroughly.

Pour in a scant ¼ cup of vodka, just enough to moisten the salt mixture. Stir, then spread the salt mixture evenly over the salmon, pressing it down. Wrap the salmon tightly in the plastic wrap.

Adapted from Sylvia Fontaine's "Homemade Lox with Vodka, Juniper, Lemon & Rosemary," *Feasting at Home* (blog), December 1, 2015.

Place the salmon in a baking dish, and set another slightly smaller baking dish on top of the fish, pressing down firmly. Pile a few cans or other weights on the top dish to weight down the salmon. Refrigerate for 24 to 36 hours (the longer the fish cures, the saltier it will get; try not to let it cure for longer than 40 hours or so).

Unwrap the salmon and gently rinse off the salt cure under cold running water. Pat dry.

Slice the salmon diagonally into paper-thin slices for serving. Garnish with dill, as desired.

Store any leftovers in the refrigerator for up to 5 days. Or freeze by wrapping it tightly in plastic wrap and putting it in a ziplock bag. When you're ready to eat it, thaw for about 24 hours.

Laurel
(*Laurus nobilis*)

Laurel, sometimes called Bay Laurel, symbolized honor and wisdom in ancient Rome. It was cut and brought into homes as decoration during winter festivals, and it was made into crowns to honor accomplished poets, oracles, warriors, statesmen, and doctors. Laurel wreaths once crowned the victors in Greek and Roman poetry competitions and at the Olympics. The circlets were made of fresh Laurel (or Olive) leaves and could also be made of gold or silver.

The Latin name *Laurus nobilis* is believed to derive from the Latin *laurus,* meaning "tree," and *nobilis,* "noble." *Laurus* may itself have come from *daurus,* which is related to the Indo-European root *deru,* "tree," in particular oak. Oak *(drys)* was sacred to Zeus in ancient Greece, but Laurel took its place in the classical period.[99]

In Rome, Laurel leaves (aka Bay leaves) were a common culinary spice. As an herb that was sacred to high Gods, such as Zeus and Apollo, and to heroes of all kinds, Laurel was held to be protective against both natural and human-made disasters. It was also said to protect against poisoning and sorcery and to shield any area where it was planted from lightning. The Roman emperors believed it would guard them against misfortunes and conspiracies. Apollo's prophetic priestesses at Delphi used it to enhance divination, chewing and burning the leaves.

Laurel was also sacred to Strenua, a Roman Goddess of the new year, purification, and health. On New Year's Day, celebrants carried her image and branches from the Laurel that grew in her sacred grove in a procession along the Via Sacra to the open space where augurs did their divinations for the new year. Family and friends would share gifts, along with laurel twigs, sometimes wound with red yarn. Each twig had seven leaves (probably symbolizing the seven known planets), and celebrants would burn the leaves as incense while asking Strenua for good health. Over time, Strenua eventually became La Befana, the Good Witch or Christmas Witch of Italian lore. She flies around on a broomstick and comes down chimneys on Epiphany Eve (the night of January 5) to deliver gifts, bless new brooms, sweep out the old year, and purify the house.[100]

This Beffana appears to be heir at law of a certain heathen goddess called Strenia, who presided over the new-year's gifts, "Strenae," from which, indeed, she derived her name. . . . Her presents were of the same description as those of the Beffana— figs, dates, and honey. . . . Moreover, her solemnities were vigorously opposed by the early Christians on account of their noisy, riotous, and licentious character.

REV. JOHN J. BLUNT, *VESTIGES OF ANCIENT MANNERS AND CUSTOMS DISCOVERABLE IN MODERN ITALY AND SICILY* (1823)

In sixteenth- and seventeenth-century England, Witches and devils were said to be rendered helpless by the mere presence of Laurel. In the Elizabethan era, from Christmas Eve to Twelfth Day, halls and houses were traditionally decorated with Laurel, Ivy, and Holly.

Throughout history, in many different cultures, Laurel was used to guard against sickness, such as plague, and was taken as tea or in baths as an antirheumatic. The leaves were used to repel insects, such as meal moths, from flour and meal, beans, grains, Figs, Raisins, and other food stores.[101]

Medicinal Properties

Laurel extract has shown anticancer effects, especially in colon and breast cancers, by triggering apoptosis (cell death). It also stimulates and regulates the menstrual cycle, eases cramps, boosts digestion, alleviates gas and intestinal spasms, relieves bloating, and increases appetite.

Laurel leaves are beneficial for colds, flu, and bronchitis. They are also antibacterial and antiseptic and ease spasms, which can soothe coughing. Externally, they make a healing antibacterial poultice for wounds, bites and stings, and rashes such as those caused by stinging nettle and poison ivy. They also can be applied to the forehead to ease a headache. To make a poultice, simmer the fresh leaves until soft or soften the dried leaves by soaking them in boiling water, then spread them on a clean cloth and apply to the skin.

The anti-inflammatory essential oil of Laurel helps with the pain of arthritis, rheumatism, gout, and aching muscles and strains when rubbed on the affected part of the body. It can also be massaged into the temples to relieve headaches and migraines and dropped into the ears to relieve earache. Rub the oil into your scalp to promote hair growth and to treat dandruff. Dispersed via a diffuser, it helps with anxiety, stress, and insomnia. (Note: For external use, add the essential oil to a carrier oil; it should comprise no more than 0.5 percent of the solution.)[102]

Specific uses include the following:

To make a hair rinse: Steep a handful of dried Laurel leaves in 2 cups of hot water, covered, for 20 to 25 minutes. Strain and let cool. Apply as a wash after shampooing to get rid of dandruff or to strengthen thinning hair. Use it as a hair rinse three times a week to combat head lice.

To improve digestion: Add a Laurel leaf (aka Bay leaf) to soups, stews, and sauces. Drink a cup of Laurel leaf tea after each meal.

To relieve joint pain: Simmer Laurel leaves in 2 cups of water, covered, for about 30 minutes. Soak a clean cloth in the warm tea, lay the hot cloth on a plate, and place the laurel leaves in the center of the cloth. Fold over the edges to make a fomentation. Apply to the affected joints for 10 to 15 minutes.

To relieve coughs: Steep 2 teaspoons of crushed leaves in freshly boiled water, covered, for 10 to 15 minutes. Strain, add honey, and drink warm.

To remedy bronchitis, fever, and flu: Steep one or two Laurel leaves in 1 cup of freshly boiled water, covered, for 15 minutes. Strain and drink. Also, soak a clean cloth in the hot tea and apply it to the chest two or three times a day.[103]

CAUTION: There is not enough data on how Laurel affects pregnancy and breastfeeding, so stay safe by using only food amounts, not medicinal amounts, in these cases. Young children should not use the essential oil, as it may cause breathing problems for them. If you are diabetic, monitor your blood sugar carefully while using this herb, as it can affect blood sugar control. It may interfere with anesthesia, so stop using it 2 weeks before a planned surgery. Do not take this herb in combination with narcotics or sedatives, as it can potentiate these medications.[104] The essential oil poses a high risk of irritation and sensitization. If you plan to use it externally, dilute it in a carrier oil, as described above.

Magical Uses

Use Laurel to enhance clairvoyance, either by burning the leaves or by ingesting them in teas and foods.

An herb of the new year and new beginnings, Laurel brings protection, purification, strength, and good health. It can be burned or asperged to consecrate a ritual area and is used to counter or break hexes and negative spells. Burn the leaves or place them in the corners of the house to protect the family. Also burn the leaves while seeking to manifest wishes and goals.[105]

Laurel at Yuletide

Laurel is an herb of fire, sacred to the Sun God Apollo. Hang boughs of Laurel in the home, and place them on the altar to honor the returning Sun. Place a branch of Laurel with seven leaves on it on the altar to honor Strenua. Give a gift of Laurel, tied with a red ribbon, to your friends and family members. Hang it on doors and gateposts to protect the home from the dark forces that may be abroad in the deep cold of winter. Burn Laurel to purify the home and as you make your wishes for the new year.

🌿 Ratatouille

Hearth Druids and Kitchen Witches who are looking for a green and red dish to grace the Yuletide table might consider the classic French ratatouille. This dish can be served with rice, pasta, risotto, polenta, crusty bread, or quinoa or paired with any kind of meat, from chicken to beef, pork, and sausages. Egg omelets and fried eggs also go well with it, as does red wine.

We live in an age when summer vegetables are easily available year-round from supermarkets, so finding the fresh ingredients should not be hard. The dish is spiced with bay leaf, and you could also lay bay leaves in a circle around the serving plate as homage to the Sun, the Sun God Apollo, and the Goddess Strenua.

Makes 4 servings

> 1 large organic eggplant (about 14 ounces), peeled and cut into 1-inch sections
> 1½ teaspoons kosher salt, plus a bit more for seasoning
> ½ cup organic olive oil, plus more as needed
> 1 large organic zucchini, sliced into ¼-inch coins
> 2 pints organic golden or cherry tomatoes (or 1 pint of each)
> 4 sprigs fresh thyme
> 3 sprigs summer savory (optional)
> 1 bay leaf
> 2 medium organic yellow onions, diced
> 1 organic red bell pepper, coarsely chopped
> 2 cloves organic garlic, peeled and sliced thin
> A pinch of crushed red pepper flakes
> 1 cup fresh basil leaves, torn
> 1 tablespoon chopped flat-leaf (Italian) parsley
> Kitchen twine, to tie up the herbs

Adapted from Miriam Hahn and Tasting Table staff's "Ratatouille," Tasting Table (website), accessed August 18, 2021.

Toss the eggplant pieces with 1 teaspoon salt and let drain in a colander for 30 minutes. This is an important step, so do not omit it!

Pat the eggplant dry with a paper towel.

Heat 2 tablespoons olive oil in a large pot over medium heat. When the oil is hot, put in the eggplant and cook, stirring often, until it is golden, 8 to 10 minutes. If the eggplant sticks to the bottom, add more oil as needed. When it's done, remove the eggplant and set it aside in a medium bowl.

Do not wash the pot! Add 2 tablespoons olive oil to the same pot and cook the zucchini until golden but not completely tender, 2 to 4 minutes. Then remove the pot from the heat and transfer the zucchini to the bowl with the eggplant. Do not wash the pot.

Put half of the tomatoes into a medium bowl. Using your hands, crush them. Season the crushed tomatoes with ½ teaspoon salt and set aside.

Tie the thyme sprigs, savory sprigs (if using), and bay leaf together into a bundle, using kitchen twine.

Heat the remaining ¼ cup of the olive oil in the same pot you used for the eggplant and zucchini. Add the onions and the herb bundle and cook until the onions are soft and translucent, 8 to 10 minutes.

Add the bell pepper and cook, stirring occasionally, until the onions and red pepper are very soft, 14 to 16 minutes.

Add the garlic and red pepper flakes and cook until fragrant, 1 to 2 minutes.

Add the crushed tomatoes, then reduce the heat to medium-low and cook until the tomatoes are very soft and the flavors have melded, 8 to 10 minutes.

Add the eggplant and zucchini and the remaining (whole) tomatoes, and stir a few times to combine. Season with salt, cover, and reduce the heat to low. Cook until all the vegetables have softened, 12 to 15 minutes.

Remove the pot from the heat, adjust the seasonings to taste, and discard the herb bundle. Top with the basil and chopped parsley and serve.

Lemon
(*Citrus limon*)

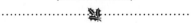

According to Greco-Roman mythology, citrus fruits were under the domain of Hera/Juno, wife of Zeus/Jupiter. They were so precious that she hid them in the Garden of the Hesperides at the western end of the world, where the Sun sets every evening. The Hesperides were nymphs charged with guarding Hera's sacred fruits; depending on the source, they numbered from three to seven. The guardians of the citruses were said to be three: Aegl tended the Citron, Arethusa the Lemon, and Hesperethusa the Orange.[106]

Lemons are native to Southeast Asia. The first citrus fruit known to Europeans was the Citron (*Citrus medica*), which came to Rome from what is now the Middle East. Citron is not very good to eat but has a fragrant rind that was used as a breath freshener. Lemons first appeared in Europe around the first century CE; by the time Vesuvius erupted in 79 CE, they were fairly well known, though very costly, and were being painted on Pompeiian frescoes.[107]

By the Middle Ages, Lemon trees were being grown as garden ornamentals in Europe. Their wood was fabulously expensive; the ultra-rich used it for making furniture. Their fruits, likewise, were available only to the wealthiest buyers and were imported mainly from Arab regions.[108] Recipes that included Lemon, of Arabic origin, were called *limonia*. The Crusaders would have become familiar with such Lemon dishes during their campaigns in the Holy Land.

From the Middle Ages through the Renaissance, banquets traditionally ended with the *boute-hors* (kick out)—the meal done, the table cleared, and wine and sweets served in another room. Generally, the sweets were spices, nuts, and fruits, candied in sugar or honey. These might include Aniseed, Coriander, Ginger, Lemons, Melons, Oranges, Pomegranates, Quinces, Almonds, Chestnuts, Pine nuts, and Walnuts, all of which were believed to improve digestion. Lemons were also made into medicinal jam.[109]

In Germanic areas, from the Baroque era to the mid-twentieth century, a Lemon might be placed in the hand of a body laid out for burial. Lemons were also carried by mourners, pallbearers, and clergy in funeral processions and cast into the open grave. The scent of Lemon was meant to protect mourners from the smell of decay and from the transmission of disease. In the Baroque age, the number of Lemons brought to a funeral showed the prestige of the deceased and their family.[110]

Christopher Columbus took the New World's first citrus seeds to

Haiti in 1493; they are said to have been Sour Orange, Sweet Orange, Citron, Lemon, Lime, and Pomelo. By about 1565, citrus trees were growing in Saint Augustine, Florida, and in coastal South Carolina.[111] For the following few centuries, citrus fruits were highly prized luxuries in colonial North America, shipped in from far distant places. Colonists enjoyed salt-pickled Lemons and candied Lemon peels.

Medicinal Properties

High in antioxidants and bioflavonoids, Lemons boost immunity and lessen the duration of colds and are also used to treat coughs and sore throats. (Most of their vitamin content is found in the white rind just under the skin, so eat that if you can!) Lemons can also be effective against flu, H1N1 (swine) flu, ringing in the ears (tinnitus), and Ménière's disease.

Lemon juice aids digestion, reduces inflammation and pain, improves the function of blood vessels, and eases fluid retention by increasing urination.[112] Drinking several quarts of lemonade daily may help prevent kidney stones.

Lemons may improve asthma and blood pressure. Their flavonoids may help lower the risk of ischemic stroke in women and may help protect against cancer and cardiovascular disease.

Externally, Lemon juice can be used as a hair rinse and facial astringent. Applied daily, it can eliminate the fungus that causes dandruff. It is also a degreaser for those with oily hair and scalp.

Specific applications are as follows:

For a cough or cold: Drink hot water with Lemon juice and honey (add 2 teaspoons of liquor, such as whiskey, for a classic hot toddy, and see the recipes on page 124), followed by a hot bath or shower and bed rest.

For a persistent cough: Mix fresh Lemon juice and honey and swallow slowly. Take freely, as needed. You can also blend Lemon juice and honey with a few cloves of Garlic to make a cough syrup (strain before administering the syrup).

To settle an upset stomach: Drink Lemon juice in hot water.

To ease constipation: Drink a glass of warm water with Lemon juice added upon rising.[113]

For a hair rinse and facial astringent: Mix 1 teaspoon of Lemon juice into 1 cup of water. Apply to the hair and scalp before showering, and leave it on for a minute.

CAUTION: Lemon is safe for pregnant and breastfeeding women when used as a food, but data on its safety in medicinal amounts is inadequate, so use with caution. Lemon juice may cause a stinging sensation in the mouth in cases of mouth ulcers. It can worsen symptoms of gastroesophageal reflux disease (GERD), such as heartburn and regurgitation. Please use fresh Lemons; bottled Lemon juice does not have the same vitamin C content. Vitamin C is sensitive to light and heat and diminishes quickly in Lemon juice if not stored in a cool, dark environment in a nonmetal container.[114]

Magical Uses

Lemons are linked to the full Moon and the Sun and can be used in both Lunar and solar rites and spells. Add a squeeze of Lemon, or float some peels, in water and leave it out under the full Moon. Use this Moon water to cleanse ritual tools, to asperge a sacred area, to anoint yourself before a ritual, and in ritual baths. Use it for baby blessings, initiations and handfastings, and other ceremonial occasions. You can also use it as a protective floor wash or as a purifying wash for surfaces in the home when you want to pull in positive and expansive energies.

Freshly cut, round Lemon slices radiate like solar wheels. Place them on the altar to honor the Sun at the Summer and Winter Solstices.

Luminous yellow Lemons carry the positive solar qualities of joy, happiness, courage, and fulfillment. Wear the peels in an amulet to dispel depression and sorrow. Give yourself a solar Lemon soak to banish the blues: Squeeze some fresh Lemon juice and add it to the bathwater; place the peels in a sachet and hang it under the faucet as the tub fills with hot water; if you live in an area where Lemon trees grow, float the flowers in your bath!

After you do a banishing or a house blessing ritual, leave behind some Lemons to attract light and joy into the space.[115]

Lemons at Yuletide

Arrange Lemon slices in a solar wheel design on the altar to evoke the returning Sun. Place Lemons and Oranges on the altar in honor of the Goddess Hera/Juno. Eat a Lemon-flavored dish or serve Lemon-based drinks after your Solstice ceremony. Dried and hardened lemon slices can be hung on the Yule tree to honor the Sun—put thin slices of Lemon on parchment paper and bake in a slow oven, about 150 degrees, turning a few times so they stay flat, for around 3 hours or until hard.

🍂 Buche au Sapin Baumier et au Citron (Balsam Fir and Lemon Log)

This decadent version of the Yule Log cake is a departure from the usual chocolate variety. Lemony and sweet, this cake carries the essence of the Sun. A touch of balsam fir brings peace, immortality, abundance, and fertility to the Yuletide table. It's a perfect treat for Kitchen Witches and Hearth Druids to serve at Winter Solstice.

You'll need balsam fir tips for the icing. You may be able to find these in the forest or anywhere Christmas tree are sold—just ask if they have any broken branches!

Makes 10–12 servings

For the Lemon Curd
1½ cups organic sugar
4 free-range organic eggs
Zest and juice of 3 organic lemons
½ cup organic unsalted butter
Pinch of sea salt

For the Whipped Cream
1 cup very cold organic whipping cream (35% fat content)
2 tablespoons organic sugar

Adapted from "Balsam Fir Tips and Lemon Yule Log," Épices de Cru (website), accessed August 22, 2021.

For the Balsam Fir Icing

¾ cup organic milk

2 tablespoons balsam fir tips

½ cup organic sugar

3 tablespoons cornstarch

2 small free-range organic eggs

1¼ cup organic unsalted butter, at room temperature

For the Cake

5 large free-range organic eggs

1 cup organic sugar

4 teaspoons organic vegetable oil

2½ tablespoons organic buttermilk

1 cup organic flour

1¼ tablespoons aluminum-free baking powder

¼ teaspoon sea salt

Organic confectioners' (powdered) sugar, for sprinkling on
the cake

Evergreen sprigs, for garnish (cedar, fir, holly, pine, or other
seasonal evergreens—but not yew, as it is toxic)

Make the Lemon Curd

Place all the ingredients into a nonaluminum pot and cook over medium heat, stirring continuously until the mixture thickens, about 10 minutes. Remove from the heat and set aside.

Make the Whipped Cream

Whisk the cream and sugar together until peaks form. Set aside.

Make the Balsam Fir Icing

Pour the milk into a large pot and bring to a boil over high heat, then remove the pot from the heat. Add the fir tips, cover, and let steep for at least 1 hour.

Strain the milk, throwing out the fir tips. Reheat the milk, bringing it to simmer.

In another pot, mix the sugar and cornstarch, then whisk in the eggs. Pour about ⅓ of the hot milk into the egg preparation and whisk well to homogenize the blend. Repeat the process two more times to incorporate all of the milk.

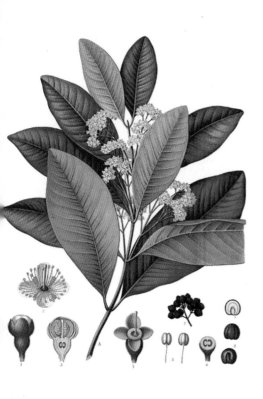

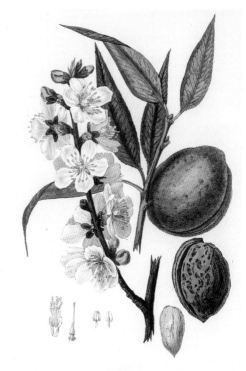

Amygdalus communis

Plate 20 (top left). Allspice
(*Pimenta dioica*)

Plate 21 (top right). Almond
(*Prunus dulcis*)

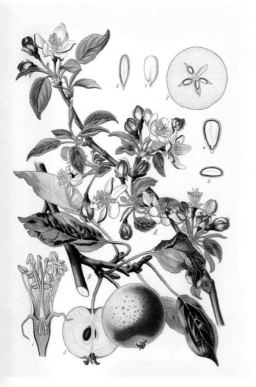

Plate 22. Apple
(*Malus* spp.)

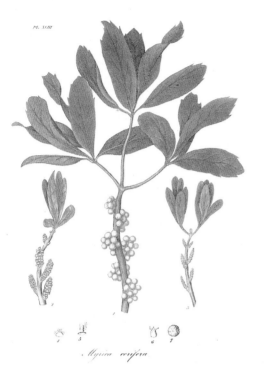

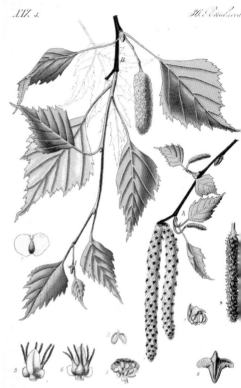

Plate 23 (top left). Bayberry
(*Morella cerifera*)

Plate 24 (top right). Birch
(*Betula pendula*)

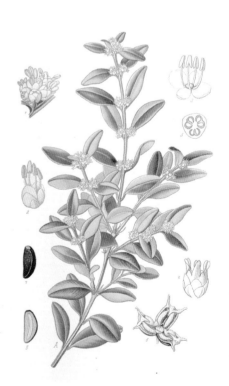

Plate 25. Boxwood
(*Buxus sempervirens*)

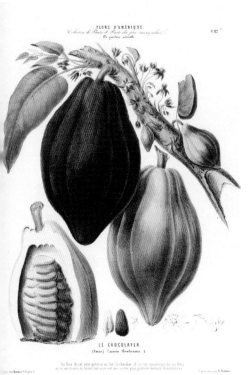

Plate 26. Cacao
(*Theobroma cacao*)

Plates 27 (lower left) and 28 (lower right). Cinnamon (*Cinnamomum cassia, Cinnamomum verum*)

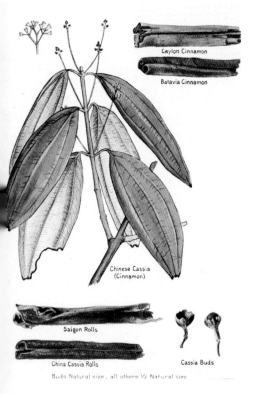

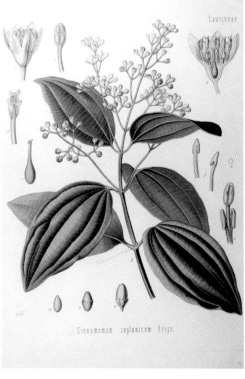

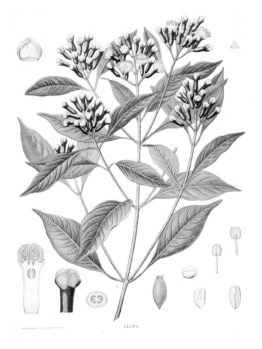

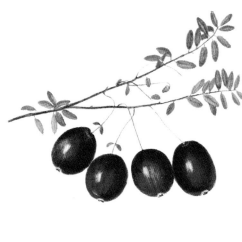

Plate 29. Clove
(*Syzygium aromaticum*)

Plate 30. Cranberry
(*Vaccinium macrocarpon*)

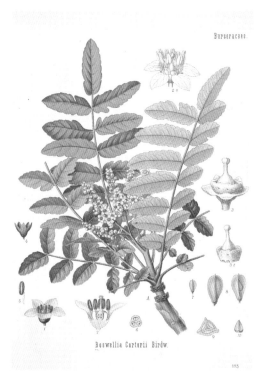

Plates 31 and 32. Frankincense (*Boswellia sacra*) and Myrrh (*Commiphora myrrha*)

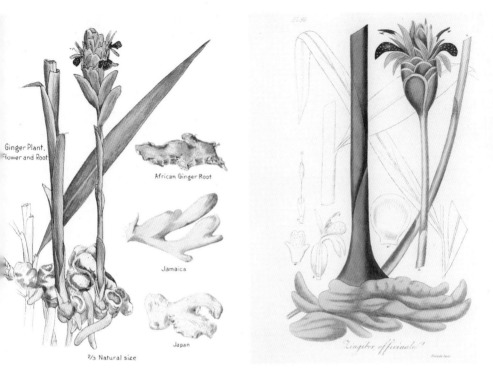

Plates 33 and 34. Ginger (*Zingiber officinale*)

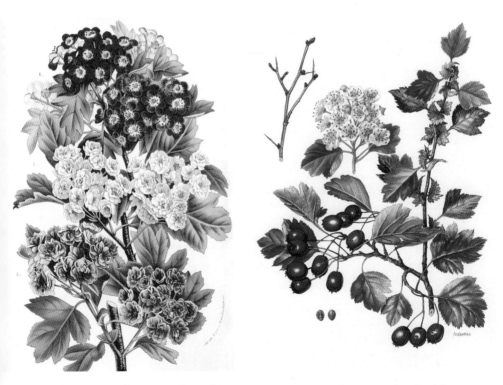

Plates 35 and 36. Hawthorn (*Crataegus monogyna, Crataegus laevigata*)

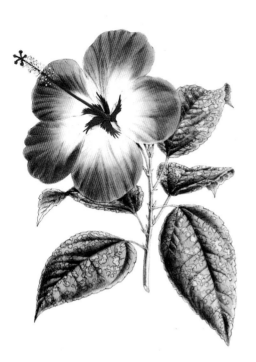

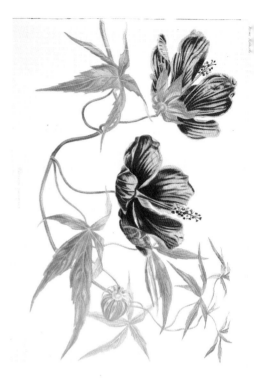

Plates 37 (top left) and 38 (top right).
Hibiscus (*Hibiscus rosa-sinensis*)

Plate 39. Holly
(*Ilex aquifolium*)

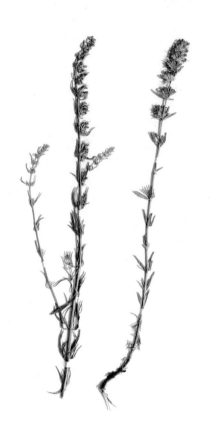

Plate 40. Hyssop
(*Hyssopus officinalis*)

Plates 41 (lower left) and
42 (lower right). Ivy (*Hedera helix*)

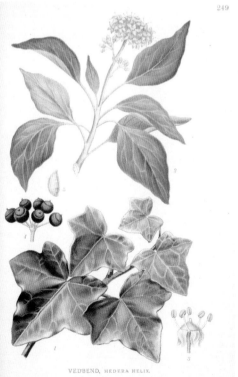

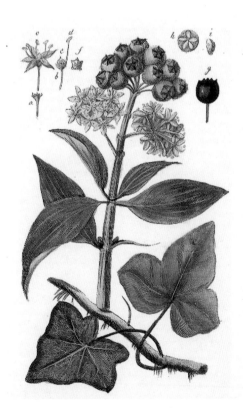

VEDBEND, HEDERA HELIX.

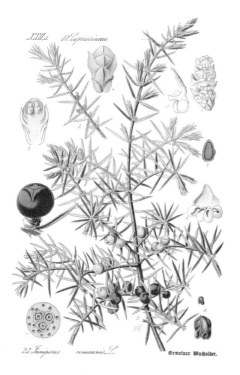

Plate 43. Juniper
(*Juniperus* spp.)

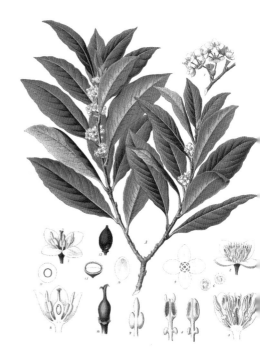

Plate 44. Laurel
(*Laurus nobilis*)

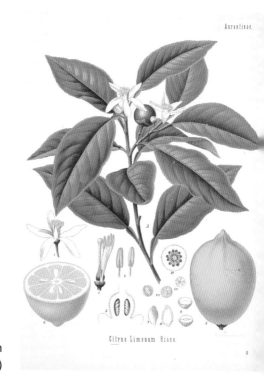

Plate 45. Lemon
(*Citrus limon*)

Heat the milk and sugar preparation over medium heat until thick and boiling. Cook for 2 minutes, then remove from the heat. Spread the preparation on a baking sheet, cover with plastic wrap, and let cool thoroughly.

Whisk the butter until creamy in a mixing bowl. Add the cooled milk and sugar preparation slowly, 1 tablespoon at a time, whisking after each addition. When the milk and sugar preparation is well combined with the butter, whisk at high speed until the blend is light and creamy.

Make the Cake

Preheat the oven to 350°F. Set an oven rack in the middle of the oven. Oil a baking sheet and line it with parchment paper.

Beat the eggs and sugar in a blender at high speed until voluminous and pale in color. Whisk in the oil and buttermilk.

In another bowl, mix the flour, baking powder, and salt. Using a strainer, sprinkle the dry ingredients on the egg mixture, then beat together until the dry ingredients are fully incorporated.

Spread the blend on the baking sheet, using a spatula. Cook in the middle of the oven for 15 minutes, or until a toothpick inserted into the center of the cake comes out clean.

As soon as the cake is cool enough to handle, slide a knife blade between the cake and the baking sheet to unstick the sides, then unmold the cake onto a clean towel. Remove the parchment paper, then sprinkle the top surface with confectioners' sugar.

Using the towel, roll up the cake into a log. Leave it in the towel for at least 1 hour to take shape as a log.

Assembly

Unroll the cake.

Spread the lemon curd over the cake, leaving a ½-inch margin unfrosted on all four sides. Spread the whipping cream evenly over the lemon curd. Then roll up the cake (without the towel this time) to fashion a Yule Log and transfer it to a serving dish.

Evenly spread icing over the log, using a fork to trace lines imitating tree bark. If you like, dust the cake with "snow" by putting some confectioners' sugar into a large strainer and shaking the sugar over the log. Decorate the edges of the plate with a sprig or two of evergreens.

Licorice
(*Glycyrrhiza glabra*)
·················· 🌿 ··················

*We're like licorice. Not everybody likes licorice, but the
people who like licorice really like licorice.*

JERRY GARCIA OF THE GRATEFUL DEAD

Though Licorice root is actually sweeter than sugar, for many centuries it was known only as a medicine. The root was most commonly chewed, taken as tea, or brewed into a beer for its medicinal effects; the soldiers of Alexander the Great were ordered to chew the roots to keep themselves healthy and hydrated. It wasn't until the thirteenth century that Licorice started appearing in confections as a flavoring agent and sweetener.[116]

In Spain, children anticipate gifts from the Three Wise Men on that night, but if they have misbehaved, they may find only lumps of Licorice candy instead.[117]

Medicinal Properties

The first documented medicinal uses of Licorice can be traced back to ancient Assyria, Egypt, China, and India. Greek scholar Theophrastus (ca. 372–287 BCE) called Licorice the "Scythian root," saying that the Greeks learned to use it from the Scythians who lived in the area of Ukraine between the Black and Caspian Seas. Theophrastus recommended the root for unproductive coughs and asthma and, mixed with honey, as a wound medicine.

The Roman author Dioscorides (40–90 CE) included Licorice in his *De Materia Medica,* advising its use for hoarse voice, chest pain, and diseases of the stomach and liver. He also recommended it for skin lesions, such as ulcers at the base of finger- or toenails. Dioscorides prescribed Licorice powder for pterygium, a web of thickened conjunctival tissue growing over the cornea that can eventually lead to blindness.

Pliny the Elder (23–79 CE) described the plant in detail in his *Natural History,* suggesting Licorice as a remedy for asthma, sore throat, ulcerations of the mouth, to combat sterility (this makes sense, as the plant is loaded with estrogen), and for kidney and bladder conditions. He cited the external use on condylomata (genital warts caused by human papillomaviruses) and genital ulcers. He also recommended powdered Licorice for pterygium.

The renowned Persian physician Avicenna (Ibn Sina) cited Licorice as a remedy for diseases of the respiratory tract and for ailments of the kidneys and bladder in his eleventh-century *Canon of Medicine*. Hildegard von Bingen (1098–1179), a German Benedictine abbess, wrote a treatise on medicines in which she reported that, together with Fennel and honey, Licorice was useful for *de cordis dolore* (angina pain).

English physician Nicholas Culpeper (1616–1654) included Licorice in his *Complete Herbal,* writing: "It is hot and moist in temperature, helps the roughness of the windpipe, hoarseness, diseases in the kidneys and bladder, and ulcers in the bladder, . . . [it] helps difficulty of breathing." He also advised its use for "raw humors of the stomach" and conditions of the kidneys and bladder. Like the ancient Greek and Roman scholars, he prescribed Licorice powder placed in the eye for pterygium, probably having learned that use from their work.

In China, the *Shennong bencaojing,* written circa 200 BCE, cites Licorice for pharyngitis, cough, palpitations, gastric pain, ulcers in the intestinal tract and sores, and intoxication by drugs and food poisoning. Early Indian Ayurvedic texts describe Licorice as useful in antidotes for acute and chronic poisonings, to improve the voice, and for viral respiratory tract infections, wound infection, surgical wounds, excessively bleeding punctures, and acute and chronic liver diseases like hepatitis.

Modern research has not shown that Licorice helps with gastric ulcers, but it has confirmed its beneficial effects on allergic and inflammatory diseases of the skin. In vitro antiviral effects were seen in respiratory tract infections like influenza and severe acute respiratory syndrome (SARS), hepatitis B virus, Epstein-Barr virus, human immunodeficiency virus (HIV), and encephalitis-causing viruses like herpes simplex virus and Japanese encephalitis virus.

For urinary tract infections, Licorice was found to be an effective remedy only when combined with other herbs.[118]

Licorice remains still a classic remedy for coughs, hoarseness of voice, and other respiratory problems and is often included in cough drops and syrups. The root tea is laxative for children and can help lower a fever. In Chinese medicine, Licorice is called "the peacemaker" because it improves the taste of herbal formulas and prevents allergic reactions. A classic herbal "triangle" to combat exhaustion and strengthen the adrenals is a combination of Licorice, Siberian Ginseng (*Eleutherococcus senticosus*), and Saint John's Wort (*Hypericum perforatum*).

For those with GERD, acid reflux, and other gastrointestinal issues, Licorice can improve digestion when taken before a meal. Look for deglycyrrhizinated Licorice (DGL) to avoid some of the side effects of the root, such as hypertension, edema, and interference with aldosterone (a kidney hormone) regulation. DGL has been shown to promote the production of mucus, which may act as a barrier to acid in the stomach and esophagus. The extra mucus allows damaged tissue to heal and can over time prevent occurrences of acid reflux.[119]

To prepare Licorice as a tea, simmer 1 teaspoon of the root per cup of water, covered, for 20 minutes. Take ¼ cup four times a day, not with meals.[120]

CAUTION: Because Licorice is sweeter than sugar by volume, diabetics should use care with this herb. Licorice has high levels of phytoestrogens and should be avoided by women with ovarian cysts, swollen ovaries, or a tendency to water retention during the menses. Hormone-sensitive conditions such as breast cancer, uterine cancer, ovarian cancer, endometriosis, or uterine fibroids contraindicate this herb. Postmenopausal women with a history of cancer or with a history of cancer in their female relatives should avoid it. Pregnant women should not take Licorice, as it can produce miscarriage or premature delivery. There is not enough data on the use of Licorice during breastfeeding, so it's probably best to avoid it at that time.

Licorice can increase fluid retention and worsen congestive heart failure, raise blood pressure, and increase the risk of irregular heartbeat. Avoid this herb if you have high blood pressure or a heart condition. Do not use it if you have low potassium. It can weaken the kidneys. As it is high in estrogen, it can worsen erectile dysfunction in men. Since it affects blood pressure, do not take it for 2 weeks before a scheduled surgery.[121]

Magical Uses

As an herb of Mercury, controller of communication and information transfer, Licorice root is, unsurprisingly, beneficial to sore throats, hoarseness of voice, and chest conditions. It is also used to get others to do your bidding, whether by burying it near their home or place of business, getting them to wear it (the oil), or having them eat or drink it. And it is used in love magic, enhancing the transmission of your will to another person. Because of its potent sweetness and high estrogen content, it is an herb of passion, particularly for women (due to the high phytoestrogen content, men who eat or drink a lot of this herb will likely *lose* potency, although it could help them to grow more hair!). Men can wear the hard little root in a mojo bag.

Wear Licorice root in a love sachet that you or your beloved carry (pink cloth for sweet affection, red cloth for passion), chew it for sexual potency, or sprinkle it in the footprints of a lover to keep them from wandering. At times, simply drinking the tea can act as a stimulant between lovers.[122]

Licorice and Anise at Yuletide

Serve Licorice tea or a Licorice-flavored treat to your beloved. Licorice root and Anise seed are close cousins in terms of flavor, though Anise is a bit more subtle. They are both herbs of Mercury and will both help to strengthen bonds between families and groups and between people and their Gods. Offer Anise-flavored cookies to the fire to send them skyward as a gift for the Gods.

Springerle Christmas Cookies

Springerle cookies are usually rectangular with a design stamped into the top. The term springerle *(SHPRING-ehr-leh) derives from the Old German* springan, *"to jump." Historians trace these sweets back to Julfest, the Germanic Pagan midwinter celebration. Animals were sacrificed to the Gods at Julfest in hopes of persuading the deities to bring good weather. But often the poor could not afford to kill any of their animals, so instead they gave token sacrifices, such as animal-shaped breads and cookies with animal designs stamped on them.*

Exchanging Springerle cookies during the holidays and at important life passages eventually came to be a traditional Germanic practice, just as we exchange gifts and cards today.

Make these cookies when the weather is dry and cold, and dry them overnight before serving. If you don't have a Springerle rolling pin (a special rolling pin with designs, like animals and wheat, carved into it), consider cutting the dough into simple animal shapes. To preserve their softness, keep the cookies in an airtight container and place a piece of bread or a slice of apple on a paper towel on top of them. When hard, the cookies are used for dunking.

> *Makes 120 small cookies*
>
> 4 free-range organic eggs
>
> 2 cups organic sugar
>
> 1½ tablespoons organic butter, at room temperature
>
> 1 teaspoon aluminum-free baking powder
>
> 1 teaspoon anise extract for baking
>
> 4 cups organic all-purpose flour (wheat or gluten-free),
>   sifted, plus extra as needed

Line baking sheets with parchment paper.

In a large mixing bowl, beat the eggs until light and fluffy. Add the sugar, butter, and baking powder and beat very fast for about 15 minutes, scraping the sides of bowl occasionally. Beat in the anise oil, then gradually beat in the flour until well mixed.

Adapted from Ann Pratt's "Springerle Cookies," What's Cooking America (website), accessed August 25, 2021.

Turn the dough out onto a lightly floured board. Knead the dough a few times, adding just enough flour to make it manageable.

Lightly flour a standard rolling pin. Use it to roll the dough into a rectangle about ½ inch thick (do not roll the dough too thin).

If you have a Springerle rolling pin, dust it with flour, then roll it slowly and firmly over the dough to make a clear design. Using a sharp knife, cut the cookies apart and trim off the outside edges. If you don't have a Springerle rolling pin, cut out shapes with cookie cutters or by hand. Place the cookies on the parchment-lined baking sheets.

Roll out any scraps of dough and repeat.

Leave the cookies out, uncovered, for at least 12 hours to dry.

When you are ready to bake, preheat the oven to 350°F. Place an oven rack in the middle of the oven.

Bake just one sheet of cookies at a time. Bake them for about 10 minutes, until the cookies are slightly golden on the bottom but white on top. If they puff up too much, gently push the bubble down. Rotate the pan from front to back once while baking.

Remove from the oven and transfer the cookies to a wire cooling rack to cool. Let the cookies stand overnight to completely dry before storing.

The longer Springerle sit, the harder they become. Right out of the oven they are crunchy on the outside but soft and tender on the inside. Keep the cookies in an airtight container for 2 to 3 weeks before using to achieve the best flavor.

Mint
(*Mentha* spp.)
·····················❧·····················

As for the garden of mint, the very smell of it alone recovers and refreshes our spirits, as the taste stirs up our appetite for meat.

PLINY THE ELDER

Mint has been used in cooking and herbal medicine since at least 1500 BCE. The Ebers Papyrus, an ancient Egyptian medical text dating to 1550 BCE, lists mint as a calming herb for stomach pains. Mint was so valued in Egypt that it was once used as a type of currency.

According to Greek lore, Minthe was a river nymph in the Cocytus, the river of wailing and lamentation in Hades. One day, Hades caught sight of her and desired to seduce her, but he was caught in the act by his wife, Persephone. In revenge, Persephone transformed Minthe into a green herb. Hades countered by bestowing on the herb such a sweet fragrance that anyone who trod upon it would instantly know its value.

Roman historian Pliny the Elder recommended wearing a crown of Mint to stimulate the mind and the soul—and to discourage lust, he added.[123] Indeed, the Greeks and Romans wore crowns of Mint at feasts and decorated the table with the herb.

Pliny also said that wild mint leaves, prepared with a mixture of salt, oil, and vinegar, were used for scorpion stings, and they were taken in wine as a drink for scorpion stings and snakebite. He recommended wild mint as a poultice for gout and lumbago (lower back pain).[124]

Mint eventually found its way into western Europe and was mentioned in Icelandic pharmacopoeias as early as 1240 CE, which recommended it as a dentifrice. Medieval monks used Mint as a breath freshener and tooth polish (as we still do today), and cheese makers, having discovered that rats and mice detested the smell, employed Mint to protect their stored cheeses.

Indigenous American herbalists used different varieties of native Mints, and when European colonists brought Peppermint and other varieties to the New World, they quickly proliferated and became naturalized. The London Pharmacopoeia of 1721 listed Mint as a remedy for sores, venereal disease, colds, and headaches.[125]

In 1670, so the story goes, a choirmaster at Cologne Cathedral in Germany handed out Peppermint-flavored candy canes to children at their living nativity scene to keep the kids occupied. The candy was shaped to look like a shepherd's crook as a reminder of the shepherds who came to visit the baby Jesus. Those first all-white candy canes were a hit, and Peppermint became a standard flavor of the Christmas season.[126]

Medicinal Properties of Peppermint

Peppermint (*Mentha piperita*) is the Mint most often used medicinally. It contains menthol, a pain-relieving agent for rheumatism, neuralgia, throat afflictions, and toothaches. It is a local anesthetic, vascular stimulant, and disinfectant. Peppermint induces perspiration and is cooling for fevers and heat stroke. It helps with heart palpitations and with congestion in any part of the body, as well as headaches, colds, and bronchitis.[127]

Peppermint leaf tea helps move gas, soothes the stomach, and cleanses the liver. The tea or essential oil benefits nervous conditions and insomnia. It is even rumored to be an aphrodisiac if taken in large amounts.

Externally, the leaves are cooling and relieve pain when used as a salve, poultice, or bath for itchy skin.

Dosage depends on the preparation:

Tea: Steep two or three leaves per cup of freshly boiled water, covered, for 30 minutes. Take up to 2 cups a day in ¼-cup doses for no more than 12 days. Then take a break for a week before resuming.

Essential oil: Adults can take 3 or 4 drops on a sugar cube dropped into hot tea, or 1 or 2 drops in a glass of water, to ease gas and stomach cramps.

Tincture: Take 10 to 50 drops in water or tea, depending on the intensity of the symptoms.

Medicinal Properties of Spearmint

Spearmint (*Mentha spicata*) has very similar properties to Peppermint. It soothes the stomach and also benefits painful urination. Spearmint and Horehound (*Marrubium vulgare*) are a traditional tea combination for children with fever.

A strong decoction of spearmint is said to cure chapped hands when applied externally.

Dosage depends on the preparation:

Tea: Steep 1 teaspoon of the herb per cup of freshly boiled water, covered, for 30 minutes. Take in teaspoon doses repeatedly.

Essential oil: Adults can take 2 to 4 drops on a sugar cube dropped into tea, or 1–2 drops in a glass of water.

Tincture: Take 10 to 50 drops in water or tea, depending on the intensity of the symptoms.

Medicinal Properties of Curly Mint and Water Mint

Curly Mint (*Mentha crispa*) and Water Mint (*Mentha aquatica*) have similar properties to Peppermint and Spearmint and may be used the same ways.[128]

> **CAUTION:** Overuse of Mint can lead to heart problems, so be sure to take a week off after 12 days of using it in medicinal doses. Pregnant and breastfeeding women can safely use Mint in food amounts but should use it very sparingly as medicine because not enough is known about its effects on a fetus or newborn. Mint leaf tea is generally safe for children, but the essential oil can cause anal burning with diarrhea and is probably too harsh for them. Peppermint oil and leaf might decrease how quickly the liver breaks down some medications, so check for interactions and contraindications or consult your health care provider before using it in combination with any drugs.[129]

Magical Uses

Burn Peppermint as incense at dusk and take the tea before bed to induce prophetic dreams. Do the same before divination, and keep some Mint leaves with your cards, bones, stones, and other divinatory tools.

Bathe in a Mint bath or use the soap and fragrance to attract money.

Mint is a powerful herb of purification and protection, and as an herb of Mercury, it is an aid to communicating with the Gods and Spirits. The Renaissance-era *Key of Solomon,* Book II, states:

> Thou shalt then make unto thyself a Sprinkler of vervain, fennel, lavender, sage, valerian, mint, garden-basil, rosemary, and hyssop, gathered in the day and hour of Mercury, the Moon being in Her increase. Bind together these herbs with a thread spun by a young maiden. . . .
>
> After this thou mayest use the Water, using the Sprinkler whenever it is necessary; and know that wheresoever thou shalt sprinkle

this Water, it will chase away all Phantoms, and they shall be unable to hinder or annoy any. With this same Water thou shalt make all the preparations of the Art.[130]*

Wear Mint in a Spirit bag or hang sprays of Mint around the house to block hexes, increase mental clarity, and attract abundance. Place a Mint leaf in your wallet to draw money. Add it to a floor wash to guard against negative energies, purify an area, and attract prosperity.

Hang Mint over the sick bed to speed healing, and place it somewhere in your work space to increase productivity and promote a fresh mental outlook. Mint can also help you find a new job or line of work.

Mint at Yuletide

Mint is a ubiquitous flavor of Christmas and Yule, probably because its taste resembles snow and frost on the tongue. Have dishes of Peppermint candies and cookies in the house. Hang Peppermint candy canes on the tree. Serve Mint tea with honey and Peppermint-flavored ice creams, cakes, and drinks at Yule to ensure abundance in the new year. If fresh Mint leaves are available, toss some into a salad or use them to decorate seasonal desserts.

🌿 Peppermint Mocha Latte

Kitchen Witches and Hearth Druids will delight in sharing this brew, filled with the power of peppermint to attract prosperity and chocolate to strengthen bonds of friendship and love. For a decadent flourish, top each serving with whipped cream and just a dusting of cinnamon.

Makes 2 servings

2 cups organic milk (cow's, almond, oat, rice, or whatever
you prefer)

Adapted from Liz and Tyler Marino's "Healthy Peppermint Mocha," *The Clean Eating Couple* (blog), November 1, 2021.

*If you can't harvest these herbs on the day and hour of Mercury (Wednesday at 8 p.m.), try to buy or barter for them at that time, under the waxing Moon.

½ teaspoon peppermint extract

1 teaspoon cacao powder

2 teaspoons maple syrup or honey

½ cup warm organic espresso

Whipped cream (optional)

Ground cinnamon (optional)

Heat the milk over medium-low heat until it is hot (if it starts to bubble, remove it from the heat immediately!). Whisk in the peppermint extract, cacao powder, and maple syrup or honey. Keep whisking until the mixture is foamy.

Pour the hot mixture into mugs, and top each mug with espresso.

Top with whipped cream and, if you like, a light dusting of cinnamon.

Mistletoe
(*Viscum album*)
......................🌿......................

Where mistletoe stays in the house, love also stays.

TRADITIONAL ENGLISH SAYING

The damsel donned her kirtle sheen;
The hall was dressed with holly green;
Forth to the wood did merry men go.
To gather in the mistletoe . . .

SIR WALTER SCOTT, "MARMION" (1808)

While the ancient Romans once decorated their homes with Mistletoe at Saturnalia, the custom of kissing under the Mistletoe most likely has Scandinavian origins. Mistletoe is associated with the Pagan Goddess Frigga, wife of Odin, king of the Norse gods. She is the Goddess of love and mother of Baldur, the gentle God of the summer's light.

Once upon a time, Baldur dreamed of his own death. This alarmed Frigga greatly, because if Baldur died so would all life on Earth: plants, animals, humans, and all other creatures. Baldur was greatly loved among the Gods, and Frigga immediately asked all beings—elementals, plants, animals, and Gods—to promise to never harm him. But the trickster God Loki saw that Frigga had overlooked just one plant: the Mistletoe.

The Gods began to play a game in which they shot arrows at Baldur, just for fun, because he was now "invincible." But Loki, ever jealous and now disguised as a woman, made an arrow of Mistletoe wood and gave it to Hoder, the blind God of winter, who unwittingly shot Baldur dead. As soon as that happened, the world went dark. As all creatures began to weep for the death of gentle Baldur, Frigga's tears fell on the Mistletoe, and they became its white berries.

Baldur was laid out on his boat, called *Ringhorn,* and his wife Nanna fell down dead at the sight. The mourners placed her body next to his, and Odin lay the magically self-replicating golden ring, Draupnir, on their funeral pyre to take with them to the Otherworld.

> *Odin laid on the pyre that gold ring which is called Draupnir; this quality attended it: that every ninth night there fell from it eight gold rings of equal weight.*
>
> SNORRI STURLUSON, "GYLFAGINNING,"
> THIRTEENTH-CENTURY *PROSE EDDA*

Baldur's brother Hermod the Swift was sent to the Underworld to beseech the Goddess Hel to return Baldur to the Aesir (the high Gods of Norse religion). Hermod rode upon Sleipnir, his father Odin's eight-legged horse, and it took nine days for him to make it through dark valleys and high mountains.

When Hermod finally got to the Underworld, Hel promised to let Baldur return to Asgard, the home of the Gods, as long as all beings in nature wept for him. And all did—except the giantess Tökk, who crouched in her cave and refused to shed a tear (some say that Tökk was actually jealous Loki in disguise). That meant Baldur could not return! But Hermod did bring back the golden ring Draupnir.

Now, it is said, Baldur cannot return to his home with the Gods until Ragnarök, also known as the "Twilight of the Gods," the final destruction of the world in the conflict between the Aesir and the powers of Hel, led by Loki.[131]

Mistletoe was also an important herb of the Celtic Druids. Pliny the Elder, writing in his first-century *Natural History,* states:

We must not omit to mention the admiration that is lavished upon this plant by the Gauls. The Druids—for that is the name they give to their magicians—held nothing more sacred than the mistletoe and the tree that bears it, supposing always that tree to be the robur [Oak]. . . . The mistletoe, however, is but rarely found upon the robur; and when found, is gathered with rites replete with religious awe. This is done more particularly on the fifth day of the moon. . . . This day they select because the moon, though not yet in the middle of her course, has already considerable power and influence; and they call her by a name which signifies, in their language, the all-healing. Having made all due preparation for the sacrifice and a banquet beneath the trees, they bring thither two white bulls, the horns of which are bound then for the first time. Clad in a white robe the priest ascends the tree, and cuts the mistletoe with a golden sickle, which is received by others in a white cloak. They then immolate the victims, offering up their prayers that God will render this gift of his propitious to those to whom he has so granted it. It is the belief with them that the mistletoe, taken in drink, will impart fecundity to all animals that are barren, and that it is an antidote for all poisons.[132]

While Pliny does not indicate the source of his account, researcher Jean-Louis Brunaux argues that it was likely Posidonius of Rhodes, a first-century BCE polymath.[133] This is, in fact, the only recorded Druid ritual we have. The "golden sickle" must have been made of bronze because gold is too soft for cutting herbs. Or the "golden sickle" may be a reference to the Moon Herself! The "white cloak" refers to a white cloth the Druids held below the tree to catch the sprigs of mistletoe as they fell, because they considered the herb too sacred to ever touch the ground. They would then divide the branches into many sprigs for use as medicine and distributed the branches to the people to hang over doorways as protection against thunder, lightning, and other calamities.

Whenever a culture weaves ceremony, lore, and magic around a particular plant, we can be sure that the herb has immense practical value. Stories and seasonal rituals were a way of handing down the knowledge that a plant was useful, from generation to generation. Mistletoe must have been an important medicine for the Celtic Druids and other ancient societies.

Medicinal Properties

Mistletoe is a tonic for epilepsy and convulsive neurological conditions, including urinary and heart conditions. I have successfully used it to help a person with neurological effects from Lyme disease, though they still required standard antibiotics to purge the organism from their system. Mistletoe is also used for treating heart conditions and to stop internal bleeding.

Mistletoe is given for very high fevers, such as those caused by typhoid; it reduces blood pressure and slows the pulse (after an initial rise). It also enhances the immune system and has an antitumor effect; a commercial preparation made from it, called Iscador, is used to shrink cancerous tumors.

Combine mistletoe with Skullcap (*Scutellaria lateriflora*) and Valerian (*Valeriana officinalis*) for nervous conditions, with Motherwort (*Leonurus cardiaca*) and Hawthorn (*Crataegus monogyna*) for myocarditis, with Blue Cohosh (*Caulophyllum thalictroides*) for irregular menstruation, and with Hawthorn and Linden flowers (*Tilia* spp.) for hypertension.

To prepare Mistletoe, steep 1 teaspoon of twigs and leaves per cup of freshly boiled water, covered, for about 20 minutes. Take ¼ cup four times daily.[134]

> **CAUTION: Be sure you are using only *Viscum album*, the common Mistletoe, sometimes called European Mistletoe. Other species are harsh and abortive and can be poisonous. Also, use only the leaves and twigs; the berries of all Mistletoe varieties, including *Viscum album*, are poisonous.**
>
> **Two leaves seems to be the correct amount for an adult dose. Anything more can cause side effects such as vomiting, diarrhea, and cramping. Frequent use or large dosages of Mistletoe can cause liver or heart damage or worsen heart conditions and liver disease.**

The preparation Iscador is generally injected, but large doses given by injection can cause fever, chills, skin rashes, pain, nausea, vomiting, allergic reactions, and other side effects. Medical supervision is necessary when injecting this herb.

Women who are pregnant should avoid the plant because it stimulates the uterus and could cause a miscarriage. There is not enough data regarding the use of Mistletoe during breastfeeding, so it is best to avoid it at that time.

Because it stimulates the immune system, Mistletoe could increase the symptoms of autoimmune diseases such as multiple sclerosis, lupus, and rheumatoid arthritis. A more active immune system might increase the risk of organ rejection, so any person with an organ transplant should avoid it. It could also worsen leukemia.

Mistletoe lowers blood pressure, so it should not be used in combination with other antihypertensive drugs and should not be taken for 2 weeks before a scheduled surgery.[135]

Magical Uses

Mistletoe grows high up in a tree, usually an Apple or Poplar, and occasionally an Oak. It gets its nourishment from the sap of the tree and has no need for soil or water. It is a mysterious plant, oriented to the Pleiades rather than the Sun, that blooms and fruits in midwinter. Not surprisingly, it is an herb of air. Hang Mistletoe in the home or burn it in the hearth to protect the occupants. Hang it in the house at Yuletide to attract and bond lovers. Hang it in a bedroom to protect against bad dreams.

Nicholas Culpeper's seventeenth-century *English Physician* recommended wearing Mistletoe around the neck as a charm against witchcraft. Wear Mistletoe in an amulet or charm if you are the target of hexes or ill-intentioned sorcery.

Mistletoe and Oak trees have a sacred affinity. Oak trees show divine favor because they attract lightning but are able to ground the stroke and survive. The lightning comes as a message from the Gods, and lightning-struck Oak can be added to any spell to magnify its power. Mistletoe found on Oak, known as "all heal," has immense magical power and can be added to any spell to enhance its potency.

Because it is a holy plant revered by the Druids and other magical practitioners, "all-heal" must never be allowed to touch the ground. Mistletoe is sacred to Frigga, Odin, and Baldur; place it on or hang it over the altar in their honor.

Mistletoe at Yuletide

As told in the story above, Mistletoe is a sacred herb associated with the Scandinavian God Baldur and with the return of the Sun at Winter Solstice. We modern people still kiss under the Mistletoe in remembrance of the tender and loving Baldur and the story of Baldur is rife with solar symbolism. Even though gentle Baldur remains in Hel's Underworld kingdom, the return of the golden ring Draupnir is symbolic of the Sun's return. Draupnir (whose name means "the dripper") has the magical ability to copy itself. Every ninth night, eight new rings "drip" from the magical golden ring, each new ring the same size and weight as Draupnir. Thus, the golden ring implies periodicity and a regular cycle, such as the ebb and return of the seasons making Mistletoe a sacred herb for the Winter Solstice and return of the sun.

Mistletoe and Yuletide have a long association, and in old England, rituals were once done with Mistletoe to ensure a healthy harvest in the coming year:

> In parts of Herefordshire . . . a mistletoe bough was traditionally cut and hung up inside the house as the clock struck twelve on New Year's Eve; the old bough, which had remained in place for the past year, was removed and destroyed in a practice called "Burning the Bush." A globe of twigs, woven from hawthorn and mistletoe, was taken out to the first field that had been sown with wheat and burnt on a straw fire. At Birley Court two globes, one inside the other, were thrown onto the fire, while at Brinsop a single ball of twigs was set alight and a man ran with it across the first twelve ridges of the field. If the flames died before he reached the end, it was considered an ill omen for the coming harvest. Afterwards, there was much cider-drinking and merriment.[136]

🌱 Yuletide Mistletoe Ball

> A 4½-inch floral foam ball
>
> Garden shears
>
> 24-gauge wire
>
> Sheet moss
>
> 20 to 30 branches of mistletoe
>
> Ice pick, skewer, or other hole-making tool
>
> 3½-inch pearl-tipped florist pins (optional), for extra
>   decoration
>
> Length of red, white, or golden ribbon

Submerge the foam ball in water for about 15 minutes, until fully saturated.

Use the shears to cut one 16-inch length from the floral wire. Cut the rest of the wire into 1½-inch pieces, and bend these pieces into a U shape.

Cover the soaked foam ball with sheet moss, securing it with the pieces of floral wire.

Cut the mistletoe into 2- to 3-inch pieces (you might need as many as 150). Poke small holes all over the ball with an ice pick, skewer, or other hole-making tool. Push the mistletoe stems through the moss and directly into the holes, continuing until the mistletoe completely covers the ball.

Place the florist pins as desired; the pearl ends will look like mistletoe berries.

Firmly bend the 16-inch length of wire into a sturdy U and insert it into the mistletoe ball as a loop for hanging. Use the red, white or golden ribbon to suspend the ball from a doorway lintel or a strong light fixture.

Remember that the berries and leaves are poisonous—do not allow children or pets to swallow them!

––––––––––

Adapted from Southern Living Editors' "How to Make a Mistletoe Kissing Ball," *Southern Living* (website), accessed August 28, 2021.

Myrrh
(*Commiphora myrrha*)
·················· 🌿 ··················

See "Frankincense (*Boswellia sacra*) and Myrrh (*Commiphora myrrha*)" on page 167.

Nutmeg
(Myristica fragrans)

....................✣....................

Nutmeg originated in the Banda Islands, east of Java, an archipelago of the Moluccas. By the sixth century nutmeg was being traded by Arab merchants in the Greek colony of Byzantium (later known as Constantinople and finally as Istanbul). The spice eventually made its way to Rome, where it was valued both as medicine and as an aphrodisiac.

Nutmeg was prized all over Europe as a medicine to ward off the plague. Fleas apparently dislike the smell, so it could actually have helped to repel those vectors of the disease. Records from fourteenth-century Germany show that it was fabulously expensive; 1 pound of pure Nutmeg was worth "seven fat oxen."[137]

When the Turks conquered Constantinople and blocked the trade routes funneling through that region, Europeans were forced to seek new avenues for acquiring Nutmeg and other spices. This was a major reason why Christopher Columbus looked for a passage to the East, and why Vasco da Gama sailed around the Cape of Good Hope to India, declaring "For Christ and spices!"

Neither of those explorers came close to the mark. Nevertheless, in 1511 Portugal appropriated the Molucca Islands and maintained a monopoly of the Nutmeg trade for a century.

In the seventeenth century the Dutch East India Company took control of the islands, enslaving the people who lived there and enforcing the death penalty on any indigenous person who dared to trade the spice. Some of the islanders continued to trade anyway, so the company ordered every male over the age of fifteen beheaded. An indigenous population of 15,000 was eventually reduced to just 600 people by the Dutch.

Just one island was spared control by the Dutch, and that one had been colonized by the English. Called Run Island, it was a source of constant tension between the two imperial powers until the English traded it for a primitive American trading post known as Manhattan.

The Dutch monopoly continued unabated until Pierre Poivre, a

French horticulturalist, smuggled out some Nutmeg seeds and successfully grew them in the French colonies of Mauritius.[138]

In an echo of its historical status as a precious spice, it was once an English Christmas custom to exchange gilded Nutmegs for luck.[139]

Medicinal Properties

Nutmeg is loaded with antioxidants and anti-inflammatory compounds that offer protection against chronic conditions such as heart disease, neurodegenerative diseases, arthritis, and diabetes, as well as some cancers. Animal studies are showing that Nutmeg reduces cholesterol and triglyceride levels, has a powerful antidepressant effect, and reduces blood sugar levels while increasing pancreatic action, at least in mice and rats. They also show that Nutmeg can boost libido and performance in males (remember that the ancient Romans once took it as an aphrodisiac!).

Nutmeg has antibacterial effects against *Streptococcus mutans, Aggregatibacter actinomycetemcomitans,* and *Porphyromonas gingivalis,* which can cause dental cavities, gum inflammation, and gum disease. In vitro, it has been found to inhibit the growth of some strains of *E. coli.* Human studies are ongoing.[140]

Nutmeg is taken as a supplement for diarrhea, nausea, stomach spasms and pain, and intestinal gas. It is also taken for treating cancer, kidney disease, and insomnia, to increase menstrual flow, and as a general tonic. However, there are not enough conclusive tests of Nutmeg as a medicinal supplement for me to give dosing guidelines. As a general rule, don't take more than 1 teaspoon (adult dose) a day.

Note: The spice known as Mace is the fibrous covering of the Nutmeg seed. The properties of Mace and Nutmeg are identical.

CAUTION: Taken in large amounts (5 grams or 2 teaspoons for a 150-pound adult), Nutmeg can cause serious side effects, such as hallucinations (and when mixed with other hallucinogens, it becomes positively dangerous). It also can cause loss of muscular coordination, central nervous system excitation with anxiety and fear, cutaneous flushing, decreased salivation, gastrointestinal symptoms, tachycardia, acute psychosis, rapid heartbeat,

nausea, disorientation, vomiting, agitation, and even death, especially if combined with other drugs and medications. Some persons have reported allergy, contact dermatitis, and asthma. Animal studies have shown that Nutmeg causes long-term organ damage when taken in large amounts.

In other words, consume Nutmeg only in amounts that would be called for in culinary use.

Nutmeg is generally recognized as safe for pregnant and breastfeeding women as a culinary spice. In larger amounts, or if taken for long periods of time, Nutmeg could cause miscarriage or birth defects. It may also cause decreased fertility in men.[141]

Magical Uses

An herb of expansive Jupiter and of the fire element, Nutmeg attracts abundance and prosperity. Carry a Nutmeg seed in your pocket for luck. Sprinkle grated Nutmeg around your home and garden to ward off ill wishes and misfortune, and hide a whole seed under the bed to ensure your partner remains faithful to you.[142]

Carry Nutmeg in a green Spirit bag somewhere on your person to attract money and success. Add it to herb spells to double the power and potency of your workings. Soak it in oil for a few weeks and use it to anoint candles and yourself to attract love and to counter hexes.

Dreaming of Nutmegs means changes are coming.

Kitchen Witches and Hearth Druids will find many ways to incorporate the magic of Nutmeg into foods. As well as its magical uses, Nutmeg is reputed to aid digestion and stimulate the appetite. Add the freshly grated spice to cookies, cakes, and other sweet desserts. Dust it over fruit salads, add it to homemade curry powder, sprinkle it on bean dishes, grate it on mashed Potatoes or Yams, and incorporate it into cheese sauces, stews, and sausages.

Nutmeg at Yuletide

As an herb of fire, Nutmeg is appropriate to use at Winter Solstice observances. Sprinkle it onto eggnog and cakes, use it in mulled wine, and apply the essential oil to candles to honor the returning Sun.

❧ "Yule in a Glass"

Makes about 10 servings

> 2 organic clementines (you can substitute mandarin
>   oranges or tangerines, but not navel oranges)
> 1 organic lemon
> 1 organic lime
> 1 cup organic sugar
> 6 whole cloves
> 1 cinnamon stick
> 3 fresh or dry bay leaves
> 1 whole nutmeg
> 1 vanilla bean
> 2 (750-milliliter) bottles red wine, such claret, Italian red
>   wine, or Burgundy
> 2 star anise pods

Wash and peel the clementines, lemon, and lime.

Place the sugar in a large pot. Add the citrus peels and squeeze in the clementine juice. Add the cloves, cinnamon stick, bay leaves, and 10 to 12 gratings of nutmeg. Halve the vanilla pod lengthways and add it to the pan. Stir in just enough wine to cover the sugar. (Hold the rest of the wine in reserve.)

Simmer over medium heat until the sugar has completely dissolved. Then bring to a boil and keep boiling for 4 to 5 minutes, until you have a thick syrup.

Reduce the heat to low and add the star anise and the rest of the wine. Gently heat the wine. Once it's warm (after about 5 minutes), ladle it into heatproof glasses and serve.

Adapted from Jamie Oliver's "Jamie's Mulled Wine," itself adapted from the *Jamie Cooks Christmas* TV series, posted on JamieOliver.com (website), accessed October 26, 2021.

❧ Wassail Bowl for Winter Solstice

A classic English wassail bowl recipe would often include ale, sugar, and roasted apples, well seasoned with nutmeg. This recipe makes a lot—enough for a large

---

Adapted from *Yankee Magazine's* "Christmas Wassail Bowl," New England Today (website), December 21, 2018.

wassailing! (See page 114 for more on that topic.) If you're planning a smaller celebration, for twelve servings use four baked apples, six bottles of ale, a half bottle of Madeira, a pound of sugar, and six eggs, but keep the spices more or less as they are listed here.

Makes 24 servings

For the Baked Apples
6 tart organic green apples, such as Granny Smith

3 tablespoons organic butter

4 teaspoons ground cinnamon

½ cup water

For the Wassail
12 (12-ounce) bottles brown ale (such as Samuel Smith's Nut Brown Ale or Newcastle Brown Ale)

2 teaspoons ground nutmeg

1 teaspoon ground ginger

½ teaspoon ground mace

12 whole cloves

6 allspice berries

4 cinnamon sticks

2 pounds organic sugar

1 (750-milliliter) bottle Madeira or cream sherry

½ cup cognac or brandy

12 free-range organic eggs, with the whites and yolks separated

Bake the Apples
Preheat the oven to 325°F.

Wash and core the apples. Pack ½ tablespoon butter and ½ teaspoon cinnamon into each empty core.

In a baking pan, stir together the water and remaining 1 teaspoon cinnamon. Place the apples upright in the pan. Bake them for about 25 minutes (make sure they stay somewhat firm and don't fall apart).

While the apples are baking, prepare the wassail.

Prepare the Wassail

Pour two bottles of ale into a large (12-quart) non-aluminium pot. Set the pot over low heat. As the ale warms, add the spices, stirring in a Sunwise (clockwise) direction. While stirring, chant the following:

I am the tool,
You are the fire.
Fill this brew
With all I desire.

Increase the heat to medium and add the remaining ale, two bottles at a time, stirring as you go. Add the sugar, stirring (and chanting) as you pour.

Increase the heat to medium-high and stir in the Madeira or sherry.

While the wassail is heating, beat the egg yolks and whites separately in two small mixing bowls; the whites should be fairly stiff but not hard.

When the wassail is hot but not boiling, pour the beaten yolks into a large heat-proof punch bowl, then fold in the whites gently. Set aside.

Add the cognac or brandy to the hot wassail (don't let it boil) and immediately remove it from the heat. (Wait until the last possible moment to add the cognac to prevent the spirits from burning off and evaporating.)

Ask a guest to help you with the next step. Pour the hot wassail slowly into the punch bowl, through the folded egg mixture. As your helper stirs the mixture, gently, in a Sunwise (clockwise) motion, consider chanting something like:

You are the sunlight,
You are the dawn,
You have the power
That goes on and on.

Remove the apples from the oven. Scoop up each one with a large spoon and float them on top of the foaming brew.

Ladle the wassail (topped with its frothy head) into ceramic mugs and serve hot.

Oak
(*Quercus* spp.)

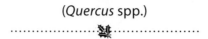

Of Nymphs and Fauns, and salvage men, who took
Their birth from trunks of trees and stubborn oak.
VIRGIL, *AENEID,* BOOK VIII (29–19 BCE)

So sacred were Oaks to the ancients that the Greeks called them the "first mothers," meaning the trees from which humankind was created. Virgil speaks of the roots of Oak descending to the Underworld in the *Aeneid.* Juvenal wrote that the human race was born from the mother Oak at the beginning of the world. Ovid wrote that Acorns were the main food of primeval humanity, while Hesiod and Homer reported that Acorns were the staple food of ancient Arcadia, the wild home of Pan, God of the forest, and his court of dryads, nymphs, and other nature Spirits.

Oak trees are considered sacred by many Indo-European cultures, including the Greeks, Romans, Egyptians, Germanic peoples, and Celts. The trees' roots go down as far into the ground as their branches are tall, making them a conduit between the Sky World of the Gods and the Underground of the Faeries and ancestors.

The Gaulish Celts did ceremonies under Oaks, such as gathering the sacred Mistletoe, and oaks were sacred to the Gaulish God of thunder, Taranis.

Oak trees were so respected as Spirits that treaties and contracts were negotiated by Druids under their branches. As folklorist Richard Folkard recounts:

> It was beneath the shade of the Oak that Druidic criminal trials were held—the judge and jury being seated under the branches, and the prisoner placed in a circle traced by the wand of the chief Druid. With the Saxons, the Oak retained its sacred character, and their national meetings were held beneath its shelter. It was below the Oaks of Dartmoor that they held their conference with the Britons, whose land they were invading.[143]

The Roman forest of Dodona was sacred to Jove (also called Zeus or Jupiter), and oracles were taken from the sound of the rustling leaves. The Romans bestowed an Oak crown of honor upon any warrior who had saved the life of a comrade in arms.[144]

The World Tree of the Prussians was an Oak, and according to Germanic lore, Faeries use openings in Oaks to create their living spaces. Hindu lore similarly maintains that Spirits use openings in Oaks to move in and out of the trees, and Scandinavian lore holds that humanity emerged from Oak or Ash trees.

In England, it was said that the best protection against Oaks haunted by Elves and Faeries was to turn your clothing inside out:

> *As in a conjurers circle, William found*
> *A menes for our deliverance: Turne your cloakes,*
> *Quoth hee, for Puck is busy in these oakes;*
> *If ever yee at Bosworth will be found,*
> *Then turne your cloakes, for this is Fayry-ground.*
> BISHOP RICHARD CORBET, "ITER BOREALE" (1647)

In many European traditions, Oak is the preferred species for the Yule Log. Its strong fire represents the waxing Sun, and burning it in the home ensures endurance, strength, protection, and good luck in the coming year.

Medicinal Properties

Oak leaves should be gathered before Summer Solstice, when their alkaloid content (which is toxic) is low. The inner bark (the thin living layer just under the dead outer bark) can be gathered from branches (not the trunk) in the early spring. Both leaves and inner bark are astringent, meaning they tend to shrink tissue, and are useful in washes for wounds, sores, varicose veins, and skin irritations and as a hair rinse for dandruff and hair loss. Make a strong tea and add it to a sitz bath for prolapse of the rectum, fistulas, and rectal tumors.

White Oak (*Quercus alba*) and English Oak (*Quercus robur*) are the best varieties for internal use (other types of Oak are too harsh and bitter for internal use but fine for external use). The tea of the leaves or decoction of the inner bark can help with bloody urine, internal hemorrhages, fever, sore throat, and mucus congestion in the lungs. You can use the tea to make an enema for piles. White Oak tea helps tone the stomach. Or soak a cloth in the tea and wrap the neck with it to shrink goiters and glandular inflammations.

Specific preparations are as follows:

For a decoction of the bark for internal use: Simmer 1 tablespoon of the inner bark per pint of water for 10 minutes in a nonaluminum pot with a tight lid. Take up to 2 cups a day in ¼-cup doses.

For an infusion of the leaves for internal use: Steep 2 teaspoons of shredded White or English Oak leaves per cup (the leaves must be gathered before Summer Solstice) in freshly boiled water, covered, for 20 minutes. Take up to 2 cups a day in ¼ cup doses.

For an enema or douche: Simmer 1 tablespoon of the inner bark per quart of water, covered, for 30 minutes.

For a wound wash: Use about 1 pound of inner bark and/or leaves (gather the young leaves before Summer Solstice) per quart of water. Steep leaves for 20 minutes, simmer bark for 20 minutes.[145]

CAUTION: Oak bark tea is generally safe for most people when taken for up to 3 to 4 days for diarrhea. Do not take it for more than 2 to 3 weeks. Overuse of Oak bark can cause stomach and intestinal problems and kidney and liver damage. Do not apply directly to the skin for deep wounds or for longer than 2 to 3 weeks.

Pregnant and breastfeeding women should avoid Oak, as not enough research has been done on its use in these situations. People with heart conditions or large swaths of eczema should avoid Oak bark washes. Do not use Oak bark baths if you have overly tight muscles (hypertonia). Avoid Oak bark if you have kidney or liver disease, a severe infection, or a high fever.[146]

Note: The tea of the spring-gathered leaves is a gentler remedy than that of oak bark. Try to use only White Oak or English Oak, internally and externally, if possible.

Magical Uses

Durable Oak trees are associated with the high Gods of the Indo-European pantheons. They attract lightning and are able to survive the blast, marking them as beings who encounter the highest divine forces and live to tell the tale. Athena, Brighid, the Daghda, Donar, Hermes, Jupiter, Odin, Perkunas, Perun, Rhea, Robur, Shu, Thor, Thunor, and Zeus are some of the Gods and Goddesses you may petition with the aid of oak. Oak is the appropriate wood for the ritual fire when calling on the high Gods and Goddesses.

Find an Oak that has been struck by lightning and use a piece of it in your herbal spells and incense. Such a tree has been blessed by the sky Gods and will add power and potency to your magical intentions.[147]

Carry Acorns in your pocket or in a Spirit bag around your neck to attract good luck and ensure fertility in your projects. Keep bowls of Acorns around your house to attract luck.

Rub your hand on an Oak on Midsummer's Day to assure yourself good health. Collect the dew from under Oak trees as a magical beauty aid, especially on Beltaine (May Day) morning.

Make an equal-armed (solar) cross with two Oak twigs bound with red thread, and hang it on the door, on a gatepost, or in a window to protect the house. Make a strong Oak leaf and bark tea and use it to wash the floors to bring protection, strength, and prosperity to the home.

Oak at Yuletide

Majestic, sacred Oak is a tree of choice for the Yule Log. Burn one in your hearth to keep light, hope, and faith alive through the darkest days of the year. For those who do not have a fireplace, drill three holes into an Oak log and place a candle into each hole.

🍂 Fallen Oak Leaf Broth

Yes, that's right: You can cook with fallen oak leaves! In fact, you can cook with the leaves of many tree species. In the fall, when the leaves begin to blanket the

---

Adapted from Mallory O'Donnell's "A Broth of Fallen Leaves," *How to Cook a Weed* (blog), October 29, 2017.

ground, consider making a fallen leaf broth. This broth is only a starter—you will keep it as a base for other additions. But why not make use of the magic of the forest?

Look for leaves in a location where they have newly fallen onto clean moss or grass, and avoid any area that is close to a roadway or is frequented by dog walkers (you can also cheat a little and pull some leaves off the trees, if necessary).

Add your leaf broth to miso soup, bone broth, mushroom soup, and more. Drink the broth like tea, adding other wild herbs such as rose hips or mint, if you like. Or make a slightly stronger fallen leaf base to add to beers and vinegars.

To begin, collect your leaves as follows:

- 50% mild, edible leaves such as beech, birch, linden/basswood, staghorn sumac, or white mulberry
- 20% aromatic leaves such as maple, sassafras, or spicebush
- 20% coniferous needles or branches such as fir, hemlock, pine, or spruce
- 10% bitter, astringent, or strong leaves such as black walnut, hickory, or oak

Soak the leaves in a cold vinegar and water bath, using about 3 tablespoons of vinegar per quart of cold water, for 20 minutes to remove any parasites. Then rinse them carefully. (For cleaning fruits and vegetables, I use plain white vinegar because it's cheaper. For dressings, soups, and tinctures, I use organic Apple cider vinegar.)

Place 6 to 8 cups of loosely packed leaves into 4 quarts of water in a large pot with a tight lid. Bring the mixture to a simmer, and simmer gently. Taste the broth often. The moment it tastes good to you, strain it carefully. Don't let it cook further or sit too long, or else the woody, bitter tannins will take over.

🍂 Festive Acorn Cake

Another way to partake of sacred oak is to gather acorns and process them into flour. The best time to do this is when the acorns first fall and are still slightly

---

Adapted from Danielle Prohom Olson, "Let Us Eat Acorn Cake! A Lazy Cook's Guide," Gather Victoria: Ancestral Food, Magical Cookery, Seasonal Celebration (website), November 4, 2014.

green. Later in the season many of the nuts will be rotten and it will take a longer time to process a decent amount.

Find two rocks to smash the nuts open; one should have a slight depression and the other rock should be flat. Place an acorn on the rock with the depression, and use the flat rock to crack it open. Drop the nutmeats into a large bowl of water as you work.

When you are finished smashing the nuts, strain out the water and put the wet nutmeats into the blender with a bit of fresh cold water. Blend the nuts into a coarse gruel. Fill glass jars halfway with the gruel and top each jar off with fresh cold water. Place the jars in the refrigerator to leach for 2 weeks, straining the water out carefully and topping off with fresh water every day.

When the acorns have finished leaching, strain the gruel thoroughly and spread it on a large baking sheet. Roast the gruel in a slow oven (about 250°F), stirring at intervals, until the acorn meal is completely dry, 1 to 2 hours.

Store the dry acorn meal in glass jars in the refrigerator until you are ready to bake, at which time you will grind the meal in a coffee grinder to make a fine, powdery brown flour.

Here is my favorite acorn flour recipe. I make this cake several times a year for special feasts and holy days.

Makes 12 servings

> Organic butter, to grease the pan
> 1 cup organic wheat flour (or gluten-free substitute), plus
>   extra for dusting the pan
> 1 cup acorn flour
> 1 teaspoon aluminum-free baking powder
> 1 teaspoon baking soda
> ½ teaspoon sea salt
> ½ teaspoon ground cardamom
> ½ teaspoon ground cinnamon
> ¼ teaspoon ground allspice
> ¼ teaspoon ground nutmeg
> 6 free-range organic eggs
> 1 cup organic olive or coconut oil
> 1 cup raw, local honey
> ½ cup organic applesauce

1 cup organic sugar

Organic confectioners' (powdered) sugar, to dust on top

Preheat the oven to 350°F. Grease and flour a Bundt pan.

Combine the flours, baking powder, baking soda, salt, and spices in a bowl.

Beat the eggs, oil, honey, applesauce, and sugar together in a separate bowl.

Combine the wet and dry mixtures and mix well. Pour the batter into the Bundt pan. Bake for 30 to 40 minutes, or until a knife inserted into the center comes out clean.

Let the cake cool in its pan for 15 minutes and then turn it out onto a rack.

Once the cake is completely cooled, dust lightly with confectioners' sugar. Serve with maple-walnut ice cream, vanilla ice cream, or freshly whipped cream on the side as a decadent seasonal treat.

Orange
(*Citrus sinensis*)
.... ❦ ....

Others, whose fruit, burnished with golden rind,
Hung amiable, Hesperian fables true,
If true, here only, and of delicious taste.

JOHN MILTON, *PARADISE LOST* (1667)

Oranges originated in southeast China, where they have been cultivated since 2500 BCE. Sweet Orange (*Citrus sinensis*) is a hybrid between Pomelo (*Citrus maxima*) and Mandarin Orange (*Citrus reticulata*). Sweet Orange was essentially unknown to Europeans until the late fifteenth or early sixteenth century, when Italian and Portuguese merchants brought Orange trees into the Mediterranean region.

Oranges bear fruit, flowers, and foliage at the same time. For this reason, they symbolize abundance, joy, fertility, and happiness in many cultures. Bridal bouquets today still often feature orange blossoms as a symbol of prosperity and luck for the marriage.

Greek mythology tells us that the precious "Golden Apples" of immortality once grew in the Garden of the Hesperides, near Mount

Atlas in Africa. There they were tended by the daughters of Hesperus and were guarded by a sleeping dragon.

One of the labors of Hercules was to obtain some of these rare golden fruits. After slaying the dragon, he picked some and took them to Eurystheus, the king of Tiryns, near Mycenae. But Minerva (Goddess of handicrafts, the professions, the arts, and war) carried them back to the Garden of the Hesperides because they would not grow anywhere else. Some modern scholars believe that the Golden Apples were actually Oranges, which would have seemed extraordinary and exotic to the ancient Greeks.

Modern traditions for Oranges continue to express the value of these fragrant fruits. In the not-so-distant past, Oranges might have been stuffed into Christmas stockings as a rare luxurious treat, and many families continue that tradition today. This tradition may have arisen from the story of St. Nicholas, who was born in what is now Turkey. Nicholas inherited a great deal of money but spent his life practicing generosity toward others, and he eventually became a bishop. (Good Saint Nick is closely associated with the gift bringer Santa Claus and may have even been a prototype for the "jolly old Elf.") One day, St. Nicholas heard of a poor man who couldn't find suitors for his three daughters because he didn't have enough money for their dowries. St. Nicholas went to the house and tossed three sacks of gold down the chimney. The gold landed in each of the girls' stockings, which were hanging by the fire to dry. The Oranges placed in stockings today may be a reminder of the saint's generosity.[148]

In Brighton, England, there was once a custom of bowling Oranges along the high road on Boxing Day (the day after Christmas). Anyone whose Orange got hit by the Orange of another had to forfeit their Orange to the thrower.[149]

Since at least Shakespearean times, pomanders have been made from Oranges; whole Cloves are stuck into the Oranges, and then the fruits are dusted (or shaken in a bag) with Orris root and Cinnamon powder as preservatives (see page 161 for instructions). The Oranges are then displayed and allowed to dry as a type of air freshener, especially at Yuletide.

Medicinal Properties

Oranges, of course, have vitamin C, but most of their vitamin content is found not in the juice but just under the skin, in the soft whitish rind. To get the full benefit from an Orange, you should eat the rind! The outer peel can be saved and dried to be added to teas.

In tea, Orange rind and peel can improve digestion, relieve upset stomach and gas, and ease lung conditions such as bronchitis. The best variety for medicinal use is Bitter Orange (*Citrus aurantium*). Sweet Orange (*Citrus sinensis*) peels also work but not as effectively, except for gas.[150]

Orange peels have other healing virtues when used on a regular basis; they can support the heart by lowering cholesterol, are antihistaminic and can ease allergies, can slow the progression of squamous cell carcinoma (skin cancer) and lung cancers, and increase metabolism and help in weight loss. A tea made from the peels can cure a hangover and help fight cavities and bad breath.

Antioxidant-rich orange peels can benefit a cold or the flu. They also support the body in getting rid of phlegm and can relieve asthma.[151]

To make a tea of the peels, steep or simmer the dried peels by themselves, or include them in other herbal infusions and decoctions as needed. You can also grate raw Orange zest onto salads and desserts as another way of absorbing the benefits (please use organic Oranges if you do this, as pesticides tend to concentrate in the peels).

The juice of the Orange has vitamin C, folate, magnesium, potassium, and antioxidants. Drinking orange juice can increase the pH of urine, which prevents kidney stones. The juice increases levels of "good" HDL cholesterol and decreases total and "bad" LDL cholesterol, as well as diastolic blood pressure. It can help reduce inflammation and prevent a number of chronic health conditions.

CAUTION: Use only organic Orange peel because conventionally grown fruits such as Oranges and Lemons are heavily sprayed with poisonous pesticides. Carefully wash your Oranges in warm, soapy water and rinse well before using the peel.
Orange peel contains synephrine, which produces stimulant

effects similar to those of ephedra. It could worsen nervousness and insomnia as well as increase risks of stroke and heart attack if taken in large amounts or for a long time.

Use caution if you have high blood pressure (hypertension) or irregular heart rhythms. Prolonged use could worsen narrow-angle glaucoma, migraine, and hyperthyroidism. In some individuals Orange peel, in medicinal doses, has caused ischemic colitis (abdominal cramping or pain, severe diarrhea with bloody stools, vomiting, and fever).[152]

The juice is very high in sugar and calories, and overconsumption of the juice can increase risk of type 2 diabetes. Try diluting the juice with water to lessen the sugar content.[153]

Magical Uses

Orange fruits and flowers embody love, luck, and prosperity. Emblematic of the round, life-giving Sun, they are the perfect ornament to place on the altar at Winter Solstice and Midsummer.

Orange flowers, fruits, and scents are appropriate for marriage rites and handfastings. The whole fruits or peels may be used in money spells. The peels may be worn in a Spirit bag to increase personal energy, success, and will.

Mix grated dried Orange zest with Cinnamon, Allspice, and Ginger (at Yule) or with Lavender (at Midsummer) to make an incense for your solar rite. Make soaps and sprays with Orange essential oil to enliven an area and increase joy and the zest for life; the scent of Orange is a natural pick-me-up when someone has the blues.

Serve Oranges and Orange-based dishes and brews to friends and loved ones to strengthen bonds of joy and to honor the Sun.

Orange at Yuletide

Place Oranges on the Winter Solstice altar as symbols of the returning Sun. Share dishes and drinks made with Oranges at your ritual. Make pomanders with Oranges and Cloves (see page 161) and use them to decorate and scent the home. Hang dried Oranges slices on the Yule tree. Put Orange slices or halved Oranges in the bird feeder as Yuletide gifts for bluebirds, mockingbirds, woodpeckers, and robins.

🌿 Mulled Hot Cider with Orange Slices

Consider the magical properties of the herbs and spices as you place each flavoring into the brew:

> *Oranges for love, luck, and joy*
> *Ginger for passion, healing, luck, and energy*
> *Cinnamon for protection, love, luck, and healing*
> *Cloves for protection from hostile or negative forces*
> *Allspice for will, energy, money, luck, and healing*
> *Cardamom for love, passion, and protection*
> *Star anise for abundance, luck, and health*
> *Apples for love, protection, fertility, and immortality*
> *Nutmeg to bring in heightened spiritual states*

(Hint: you can tie up the spices in a muslin bag or cheesecloth so no straining is required. You can also make this in a slow cooker or crock pot.)

Makes 8 servings

> ½ gallon hard or organic sweet cider
> 3 slices organic orange, plus a few more for garnish
> 1-inch piece of fresh organic ginger, sliced into thin coins
> 1 cinnamon stick (plus a bit more for garnishing)
> 5 whole cloves
> 5 whole allspice berries
> 1 tablespoon whole cardamom pods
> 1 whole star anise, plus more for garnish
> Sliced organic apples, for garnish
> Grated nutmeg, for garnish
> Honey or maple syrup (optional), to taste

Adapted from Colleen Codekas's "Mulled Hard Cider: Warm Spiced Apple Drink for Fall," *Grow Forage Cook Ferment* (blog), December 4, 2020.

Pour the cider into a large nonaluminum pot over medium heat. Add the orange slices and the ginger, cinnamon stick, cloves, allspice, cardamom, and star anise. Heat until barely simmering, then reduce the heat to low and keep the cider at a low simmer for at least 20 minutes.

When you're ready to serve, scoop or strain out the orange slices and spices (or just pull out the muslin bag, if that's what you are using). Ladle the mulled cider into individual mugs. Garnish each mug with a fresh apple or orange slice and freshly grated nutmeg, plus a small piece of cinnamon stick and a star anise, if desired.

🌱 Rosemary Champagne Cocktail with Blood Orange

Along with energizing orange, this drink features magical rosemary, an herb of fire that wards off evil forces, purifies the mind and psyche, and helps with past life recall.

Makes 2 servings

For the Rosemary Syrup
4 cups water
4–8 sprigs fresh rosemary
2 cups raw, local honey

For the Beverage
2–4 tablespoons rosemary syrup
4 tablespoons organic blood orange juice (or any other citrus juice)
Champagne (or sparkling water as a nonalcoholic substitute)
Rosemary sprigs and blood orange slices, for garnish

Make the Syrup

Combine the water and rosemary sprigs in a pot. Bring to the boil, then immediately reduce the heat and simmer for 15 to 20 minutes. Remove from the heat and let cool to room temperature.

Adapted from Colleen Codekas's "Rosemary Champagne Cocktail with Blood Orange," *Grow Forage Cook Ferment* (blog), December 4, 2020.

Remove the rosemary sprigs. Stir in the honey.

Transfer the syrup to a glass jar with a tight lid and store in the refrigerator until ready to use. It will keep for up to 1 month.

Make the Libation

Place 1 to 2 tablespoons of rosemary syrup in each glass. Add the orange juice and stir Sunwise (clockwise). Chant as you do this:

> We are one with the infinite Sun
> Forever and ever and ever.

Top off each glass with champagne (or sparkling water), tilting the glass as you pour to minimize excess bubbles. Garnish each glass with a rosemary sprig and an orange slice.

Pine
(*Pinus* spp.)
and Other Conifers

Few are altogether deaf to the preaching of pine trees. Their sermons on the mountains go to our hearts; and if people in general could be got into the woods, even for once, to hear the trees speak for themselves, all difficulties in the way of forest preservation would vanish.

JOHN MUIR, IN A SPEECH AT THE ANNUAL MEETING
OF THE SIERRA CLUB, NOVEMBER 23, 1895

Who hasn't felt the magic of sitting near a Christmas tree festooned with lights and shimmering decorations? Evergreen pines have held sacred associations across many cultures. Pagans have decorated their homes with Pine boughs at the Winter Solstice for millennia. The ancient Romans used evergreens such as Pine to welcome in the new year, as symbols of immortality and life carrying on through the depths of winter. The ancient Persian legend of the Grove of Eridhu featured a Black Pine tree, the World Tree at the center of the Earth. Its roots were of white crystal, and its foliage reached all the way to the heavens. The Persians referred to it as the Great Mother.

The Greek Goddess Cybele was worshipped in forests, where her devotees ran all night, clashing symbols, singing, playing pipes, and burning
torches in a frenzied commemoration of Cybele's loss of her lover Attis.
Attis had died at his own hand beside a Pine tree, his soul transmigrating
into the tree and his spilled blood turning into Violets at its base. Cybele,
brokenhearted, begged Zeus to return Attis to life, but he refused her
request. To ease her sorrow, Zeus decreed that Attis's body would never
decay, his hair would always keep growing, and his fingers would forever
move. In this way, evergreen Pine became a symbol of eternal life, while
Violets became a symbol of spring and eternal hope.[154]

The earliest recorded Christmas tree was erected in 1441, in Tallinn,
Estonia, by the Brotherhood of Blackheads, a military-commercial association of merchants, ship owners, and foreigners. The group decorated
a tree for the holiday festivities in their House of the Brotherhood, and
on the last night they took the tree to the town square, where members and townsfolk danced around it before it was finally set on fire.
Admittedly, today we don't know whether the "tree" was an actual
Spruce (*Picea* spp.) or a wooden pyramid decorated with paper shapes,
flowers, fruits, and toys.

The tradition of public Christmas trees took root. Records show
that in 1444, a Christmas tree was set up in London, covered in Ivy
and Holly, for the pleasure of the public, while in 1510, in Latvia, an
evergreen tree was decorated with Roses, carried to the town square,
and burned as a Yuletide celebration.

The practice of setting up Christmas trees in the home appears to have
originated later, perhaps in Strasburg, Germany, in the early 1600s, where
decorations included "roses cut of many-colored paper, apples, wafers, gilt,
sugar."[155] Later, the "bride's tree" tradition developed in Bavaria, where
magical objects were hung on the Christmas tree to ensure a happy marriage. Other standard ornaments might include the following:

- An angel for divine guidance
- Birds for joy and happiness
- Birds in the nest for confidence
- Fish for many blessings

- Flower baskets for beauty and good luck
- Fruit baskets for generosity and abundance
- Hearts for true love and a loving home
- Houses for shelter and protection
- Pine cones for motherhood and fertility
- Rabbits for hope and harmony with wild nature
- Roses for faithfulness in love
- Teapots for hospitality
- Saint Nicholas for goodwill
- Carrots for success in cooking
- Stars for guidance
- Boats so the couple might successfully sail the waters of life
- Colored balls as symbols of the many spheres of life
- Chains and garlands symbolizing cohesiveness and working together
- Lights for the returning Sun
- Grapes as symbols of friendship and good cheer
- Bells to symbolize joy

The last ornament to be hung was traditionally a glass pickle. The child who found it was rewarded for their diligence in searching, and finding the pickle was said to ensure good luck in the coming year.[156]

Queen Charlotte of England had a Yew tree decorated with toys and sweets at Windsor Castle in 1800, and when Queen Victoria married Albert of Saxe-Coburg-Gotha in 1840, the Christmas tree finally became a fashionable household fixture in Europe. It happened because Prince Albert, who loved everything about a traditional German Christmas, made a point of sending Christmas trees to schools and army barracks. Also, a widely shared engraving of the royal family with their decorated tree made the rounds in 1848 and the trees became the rage with British families.[157] Eventually, German immigrants brought the tradition to the United States and Canada.

The earliest household Christmas trees were small and without decoration. They sat on a tabletop or were hung from the rafters. By the nineteenth century, they were becoming larger and decorations, including candles, were being used. (Today, real candles are still favored by many Europeans.)

In the Iroquois (Haudenosaunee) Confederacy tradition, White Pine (*Pinus strobus*) is the Tree of Peace. A thousand years ago, so the story goes, five Native American nations were at continuous war until a prophet, known as the Peacemaker, and Hiawatha met with the leaders of those nations by the shores of Lake Onondaga. The Peacemaker told the warriors to uproot a large White Pine and place their weapons of war into the hole left by the roots. Then the tree was replanted. This was the first "burying of the hatchet" to ensure peace.

As the Indigenous Values Initiative of the Onondaga Nation describes it:

> The Peacemaker said that the Chiefs will be standing on the earth like trees, deeply rooted in the land, with strong trunks, all the same height (having equal authority) in front of their people, to protect them, with the power of the Good Mind–not physical force. On top of the tree sits an eagle who serves as an ever-vigilant protector of the Peace.[158]

White Pine was chosen for the ceremony because of its growth pattern—it grows in a circle, like the hoop of life. Its branches bend, symbolizing humility and a willingness to compromise. It has a tacky sap, symbolizing cohesiveness and the people sticking together. The needles grow in bundles of five, like the human family, and the bundles grow on a twig, symbolizing the clan. All the twigs come together in the same trunk, symbolizing the nation. The eagle that sits on top of the tree is the "one who sees far" and understands the consequences of things, like the sadness and terror of perpetual warfare.

Medicinal Properties

Conifers are anti-inflammatory and are mildly effective against bacteria and fungi. The inner bark, sap, and needles of conifers can be made into a fomentation or poultice for wounds or a plaster for rheumatic pain and sore muscles. You can apply the fresh sap directly to a wound as a dressing.

Pine resin is obtained by harvesting the dripping sap from the trees or by tapping them. The resinous gum can be chewed to relieve a sore throat or spread on a bandage to encourage wound healing. If dried and powdered, the resin can be blown through a straw into the back of the mouth to reach an infected throat.

Pine resin can be mixed and melted with beeswax and spread on a cloth to make a plaster for sciatica, sore muscles, and lung complaints.

Healing salves and ointments can be made from beeswax, vegetable oil, and pine resin. These are useful for treating eczema and psoriasis and for wound healing (do not apply to deep cuts). Melt a ½ cup of pine resin gathered from the tree in a double boiler over low heat with ¼ cup of oil (olive, almond, jojoba, coconut oil, etc.) until the pine resin melts. Then strain and return the liquid to the pot. Add ½ ounce grated beeswax and simmer gently until the bee's wax melts. Pour into jelly jars, allow to cool and when hard, cap. Store in a cool dark place.

The needles, green cones, and inner bark of the twigs can be gently simmered or baked in oil in a low oven (at about 200°F) to make a massage oil.

Pine twigs, green cones, and sprigs of needles can be simmered for about 30 minutes to make a strong tea that, when added to bathwater, will be especially beneficial to the elderly. The bath is stimulating to the skin, strengthens blood vessels, and helps with kidney and bladder complaints. The hot Pine bath should be followed by a quick cold shower.

Some Native American peoples used Black Spruce (*Picea mariana*), young tips of Hemlock (*Tsuga canadensis*), and White Pine as antiscorbutics. They also used the inner bark of White Pine twigs in cough remedies.

In the South of the United States, a spring tonic was once made consisting of Spruce tips simmered in molasses.

A tea of the inner bark and young twigs of Hemlock benefits bladder and kidney problems and can be used as an enema for diarrhea. It also makes a wash for wounds and a gargle for throat and mouth issues.

The inner bark and twigs of Balsam Fir (*Abies balsamea*) can be simmered with four times their weight of glycerin and honey to make a syrup useful for treating bladder conditions and kidney complaints, lung conditions, fever, and rheumatic pains. The dose is 1 teaspoon, four times a day.

Balsam fir resin is used to make liniments for muscle and joint pain.[159]

There is a seasonality to the medicinal use of conifers. White Pine is the gentlest internal remedy for coughs, colds, and lung congestion and can be used in all seasons. For other conifers, use the new spring growth.

The dosage depends on the preparation:

Needle tea: Steep 2 teaspoons of needles per cup of freshly boiled water, covered, for 30 minutes. Take ¼ cup four times a day.

Bark tea: Steep 1 teaspoon of the inner bark or new growth of the branch tips per cup of freshly boiled water, covered, for 30 minutes. Strain and take in tablespoon doses.

Tincture: Take 2 to 10 drops in water or tea, depending on the severity of the illness.[160]

> **CAUTION: Please be very sure of the species of conifer you are using. Do not use Yew (*Taxus* spp.) as medicine; it is poisonous. These varieties are safe: Spruces (*Picea* spp.), Douglas Fir (*Pseudotsuga menziesii*), Firs (*Abies* spp.), Hemlocks (*Tsuga* spp.), Pines (*Pinus* spp.), and Redwood (*Sequoia sempervirens*). There is not enough evidence to say whether the medicinal use of Pine and other conifers is safe for breastfeeding and pregnant women. Some people are allergic to the pollen.[161]**

Magical Uses

> *From its lofty position above the tops of most other trees, the pine reminded ancient peoples of the importance of taking the overview, encouraging objectivity and farsightedness.*
> JANE GIFFORD, *THE WISDOM OF TREES*

Burn Pine needles, alone or mixed with Juniper and Cedar needles, to scent and purify the home and draw in peace. The smoke will also send evil back to the sender. Throw a pinch of Pine into the hearth to dispel evil, and burn Pine needles before divination.

Carry conifer cones in a Spirit bag as a fertility charm (tiny green Hemlock cones are ideal for this).

Place freshly cut Pine boughs in or on top of a coffin as an emblem of immortality. (In Orthodox Jewish funerals the only permissible wood for a coffin is pine.)[162]

Wash the floors with Pine tea to repel negativity and ward off illness (even commercial Pine Sol works for this!).

Place Pine boughs on the altar to attract peace and to protect the area. Hang a Pine bough over the sick bed for health, and place one over the front door to bring joy to all who come and go.

Pine at Yuletide

A Yuletide Pine tree can become a magical talisman in the home. Special ornaments can be crafted that reflect your intentions in the coming year. And as mentioned in the chapter on Lemons (see page 213) slices of citrus fruits can be dried and hung from ribbons all over the tree in honor of the strengthening Sun.

Hang bunches of Pine or a Pine wreath on the door to bring peace to the house. Lay Pine boughs along lintels and the fireplace. Simmer fresh Pine branches with Orange slices, Cinnamon sticks, Star Anise, and Apple slices to scent the home.

The evergreen Advent wreath is thought to have been invented by Lutheran pastor Johann Hinrich Wichern in the early 1800s. The idea was to light one candle affixed to the wreath each week in the four weeks leading up to Christmas. Follow this custom in the weeks leading up to the Winter Solstice using golden yellow candles as another way to honor the returning Sun.

🌿 Conifer Crème Brûlée

First, make sure you have identified an edible conifer, harvested in the correct season; see the discussion above. Each has a unique flavor. Never use yew, as it

Adapted from Susan and Aaron von Frank's "Recipe: Christmas Tree Crème Brûlée (Made w/ Conifer Needles)," Tyrant Farms (website), November 13, 2021.

is toxic, and do not use needles from commercially grown Christmas trees, as they are heavily sprayed with pesticides. Gather fresh needles from the species you are using directly from a tree in your own yard or in a forest.

Makes 6 servings

For the Conifer Cream

¼ cup fresh conifer needles (fir, spruce, redwood, Douglas fir, pine, or hemlock)

1 cup organic whipping cream

For the Conifer Sugar

¼ cup conifer needles

1 cup organic white sugar

For the Crème Brûlée

3 free-range organic egg yolks

½ cup organic white sugar

1 teaspoon pure vanilla extract

2 cups Conifer Cream

A pinch of salt

6 tablespoons Conifer Sugar

Make the Conifer Cream

Combine the conifer needles with ¼ cup cream in a blender. Blend until the mixture is too thick to continue, then add more cream. Repeat the process until you have used all the cream and the mixture has a whipped cream consistency.

Next, follow either the cold infusion or hot infusion method.

For a cold infusion: Scoop the cream into a glass jar, cover, and refrigerate for 3 days. Stir for 1 minute twice a day to break down any bubbles and fully extract the pine flavor. On day 3, warm the cream in a pot over a very low heat until it returns to a liquid, about 5 minutes. Strain through cheesecloth or a wire mesh strainer to remove all the needles.

For a hot infusion: Scoop the cream into a pan over medium heat. Warm, stirring or whisking every few minutes to prevent sticking, for about 30 minutes. (If it begins to bubble over, remove the pan from the heat immediately.) Then remove from the heat. Strain through cheesecloth or a wire mesh strainer to remove all the needles.

Make the Conifer Sugar

Place half of the conifer needles (2 tablespoons) and one-quarter of the sugar (¼ cup) in a coffee grinder. Grind until very smooth and green and then scrape into a bowl.

Repeat with the remaining 2 tablespoons of needles plus another ¼ cup sugar.

Place the remaining ½ cup of sugar into the grinder and pulse to absorb any leftover flavor. Add to the bowl with the rest of the conifer sugar and stir well.

Store the sugar in a glass jar with a tight lid in the refrigerator for up to 6 months (the color will gradually turn brown, but the sugar will still be edible).

Make the Crème Brûlée

Preheat the oven to 325°F. Arrange six empty ramekins in a large, deep baking dish.

In a large bowl, whisk together the egg yolks, white sugar, and vanilla. Set aside.

Combine the cream and salt in a pan over medium heat. Warm, stirring occasionally, until the cream begins to simmer, then immediately remove the pan from the heat (don't let the cream boil).

While you're heating the cream, bring a quart of water to a boil for the water bath. Keep it hot.

Slowly pour the hot cream into the egg yolk mixture, whisking vigorously all the while to prevent the egg yolks from scrambling or forming chunks.

Pour the custard mixture evenly into the six ramekins. Pour the hot water into the baking dish until it's rises about halfway up the side of the ramekins. Using oven mitts, carefully transfer the baking dish to the oven.

Cook for 30 to 45 minutes, depending on size of the ramekins. The custard is done when it's firm on the sides but still jiggly in the center.

Remove the ramekins from the oven and let them cool on a baking rack. When they're cool, cover them and put in the refrigerator to chill for 4 to 24 hours.

When you're ready to serve them, pull the ramekins out of the refrigerator. Sprinkle 1 tablespoon of Conifer Sugar over the custard in each ramekin. Tap and swirl each ramekin to spread the sugar until it forms an even coating.

To caramelize the sugar, you can use either a kitchen torch or your oven broiler.

Kitchen torch method: Hold the torch about 6 inches above the surface of the sugar. Aim the flame at one point on the inside edge of ramekin. As the sugar begins to boil and darken, move to the next spot in a slow, steady circling motion around the ramekin, from the outside in, until the entire surface is adequately caramelized.

Oven broiler method: Turn on the broiler and move an oven rack to either the first or second shelf. Place the ramekins in same baking dish you cooked them in, but this time fill the dish with cold water to help prevent the custard from heating while the sugar caramelizes. When the broiler is hot, put the baking dish in the oven. Turn on the oven light and carefully watch the sugar on the custards, since it will go from uncooked to caramelized very quickly.

Serve immediately!

You can use any leftover Conifer Sugar to coat a cocktail glass, incorporate it into sugar cookie recipes, add to cups of tea, and so on.

Poinsettia
(*Euphorbia pulcherrima*)

.... ❧ ....

Poinsettias grow wild in the tropical dry forests of Mexico and Guatemala and were once used by the Aztecs as medicine and to make a red dye. The Aztecs called Poinsettia *cuetlaxochitl* (brilliant flower), and the Mayans referred to it as *k'alul wits* (ember flower). The "petals" may be white to pink or brilliant red. (The "petals" are actually leaves, while the flower is the tiny yellow bud in the center of each leaf cluster.)

The Aztecs regarded all flowers, with their fragrance and beauty, as sacred gifts from the divine. For them, the red Poinsettia was symbolic of the purity of the sacrifice warriors made for their people, and of the reincarnation of fallen warriors, who would be reborn as the hummingbirds and butterflies that drink the nectar from these flowers.

The Aztecs also honored the sacred blood sacrifice of motherhood and childbirth and held the red Poinsettia as sacred to mothers as well.[163] The plant's latex, of course, resembles mother's milk.

In the seventeenth century, Franciscan monks in Mexico began incorporating the red flowers into their Christmas decorations, declaring that the shape of the flower echoed that of the Star of Bethlehem and the red color the blood of the wounded Christ. (Given the associations of purity, sacrifice, and rebirth that indigenous peoples already had with this plant, it's easy to see why Franciscan friars would have wanted to co-opt it for their Christmas observances.) A legend was grafted onto the plants telling of a young girl, named Pepita, who wanted to bring a gift for the baby Jesus to her church. Because she was very poor, all she could do was to pick a small bouquet of roadside weeds, which made her feel embarrassed when she walked into the chapel.

Approaching the altar, she knelt and placed her bouquet of weeds at the base of the nativity scene, and the weeds immediately burst into red flowers. Everyone who saw declared it a miracle, and from that day on, the bright red flowers of the Poinsettia became known as the *Flores de Noche Buena,* or Flowers of the Holy Night.

That legend, and the red flowers, remained an obscure Mexican tradition until Joel Roberts Poinsett, a botanist, cofounder of the Smithsonian Institution, and first U.S. ambassador to Mexico, saw the plants and shipped some back to his home in South Carolina. There he propagated and distributed the Poinsettias, giving them to friends as Christmas gifts. A Pennsylvania nursery then began cultivating the plants and an intense commercial campaign popularized the modern use of Poinsettias as Christmas decorations in the United States.[164]

Medicinal Properties

Despite popular belief, the plant is not terribly toxic, though it may cause nausea, vomiting, diarrhea, eye irritation, allergic reactions, or skin rash in some humans and pets.

In traditional Mexican medicine, the latex of the stems is placed on warts to remove them. Women who are breastfeeding lick the latex or place it on their breasts to promote the production of breast milk. The latex can also be applied topically as a depilatory.

A fomentation made from a tea of the flowers, with Lemon juice, is applied topically to ease muscle, joint, and bone pain. The crushed flowers can be applied externally to help heal conjunctivitis. Internally, a flower petal tea can be taken to remedy respiratory conditions like coughs, colds, sore throats, and bronchitis.

Poinsettia leaves contain anthocyanins, which have anti-inflammatory and anticarcinogenic properties and are helpful in preventing cardiovascular and neurodegenerative diseases. Women who are breastfeeding may eat the leaves (raw or cooked) to promote breast milk. The leaves can also be prepared as a soothing poultice; a cool poultice is helpful for inflammations, and a warm one for bone and muscle contusions.[165]

> **CAUTION: Do not use commercially grown Poinsettias for medicine as they will be contaminated with pesticides. If you can keep a Poinsettia alive in your home for 3 years and only use organic plant food and natural bug prevention methods, then you can think about using it herbally.**

The latex can cause blisters and dermatitis and irritate the eyes in some individuals. It can cause vomiting, diarrhea, and nausea when eaten or taken internally. The plant may cause abortion, so pregnant women should probably avoid it. Persons with stomach ulcers, irritable bowel syndrome, or Crohn's disease are advised not to use it.[166] Also, Poinsettia is mildly toxic to dogs and cats.

Magical Uses

As an herb of the Sun and of fire, Poinsettia in the home radiates positivity, courage, joy, strength, generosity, transformation, and leadership.

Decorate the altar with Poinsettias to honor a fallen warrior or a new mother.

Poinsettia at Yuletide

Poinsettia flowers radiate like stars, and at Yuletide we welcome the return of our own nearest star, the Sun. Use flaming red Poinsettias to decorate the Solstice altar in honor of the Sun's rebirth.

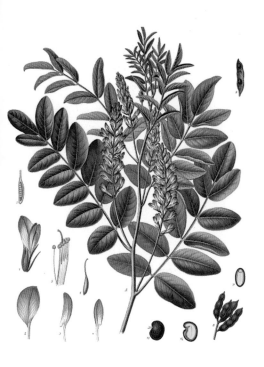

Plate 46. Licorice
(*Glycyrrhiza glabra*)

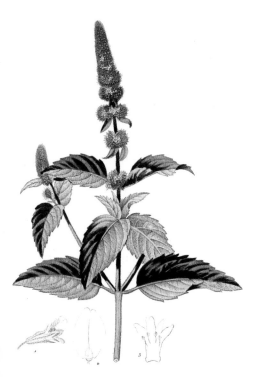

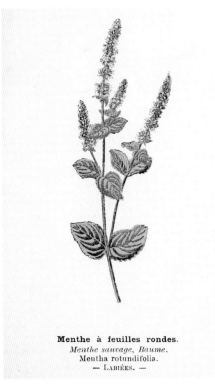

Menthe à feuilles rondes.
Menthe sauvage, Baume.
Mentha rotundifolia.
— Labiées. —

Plates 47 and 48. Mint (*Mentha* spp.)

Plate 49. Mistletoe
(*Viscum album*)

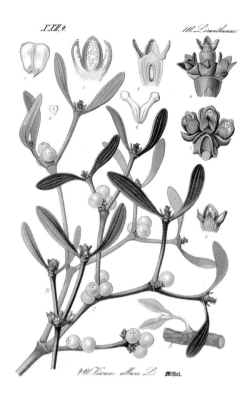

Plates 50 (lower left) and 51 (lower right).
Nutmeg (*Myristica fragrans*) and
Other Yuletide Spices

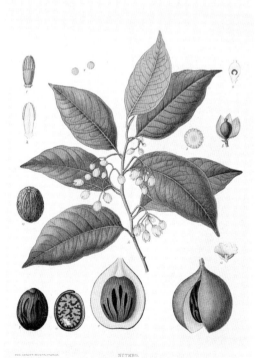

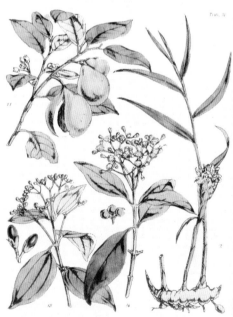

11 Nutmeg Plant   12 Ginger Plant   13 Cinnamon Plant   14 Allspice Plant

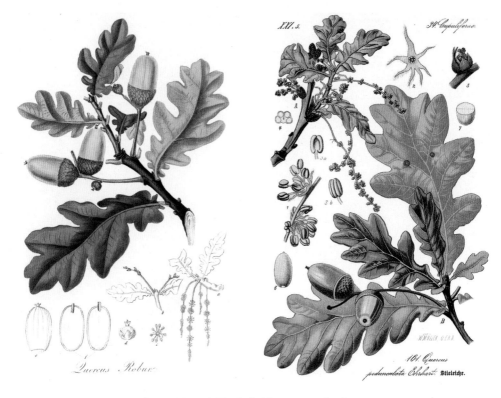

Plates 52 and 53. Oak (*Quercus robur*)

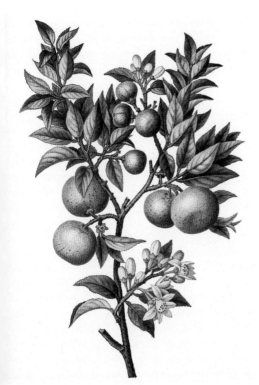

Plate 54. Orange
(*Citrus sinensis*)

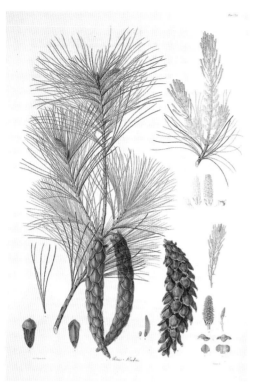

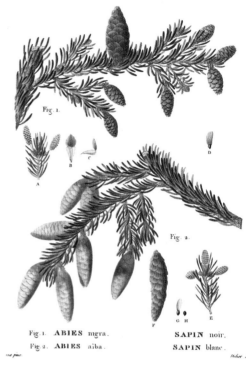

Fig. 1. **ABIES** nigra.   **SAPIN** noir.
Fig. 2. **ABIES** alba.   **SAPIN** blanc.

Plates 55, 56, and 57. Pine and Other Conifers—Eastern White Pine (*Pinus strobus*), Black Spruce (*Abies nigra*), Silver Fir (*Abies alba*), Firs (*Abies* spp.)

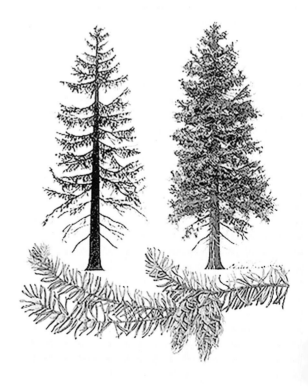

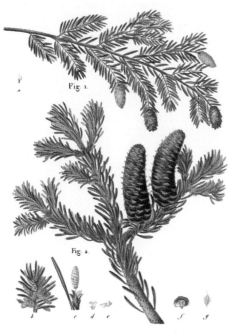

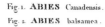

Fig. 1. **ABIES** Canadensis.   **SAPIN** du Canada.

Fig. 2. **ABIES** balsamea.   **SAPIN** Baumier.

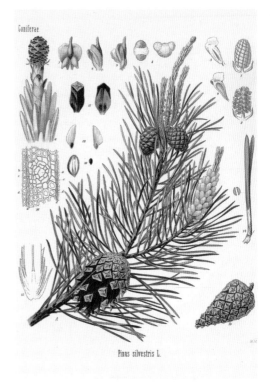

Pinus silvestris L.

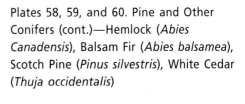

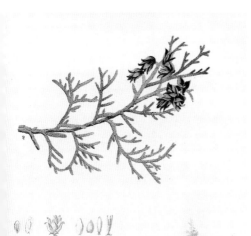

Plates 58, 59, and 60. Pine and Other Conifers (cont.)—Hemlock (*Abies Canadensis*), Balsam Fir (*Abies balsamea*), Scotch Pine (*Pinus silvestris*), White Cedar (*Thuja occidentalis*)

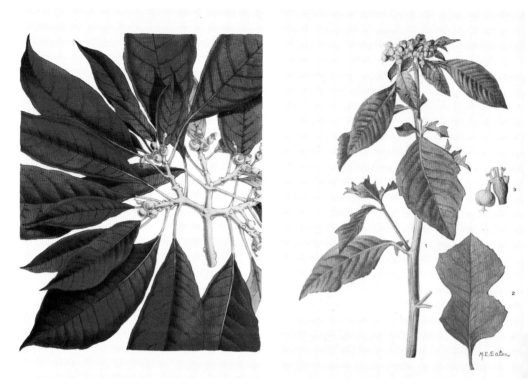

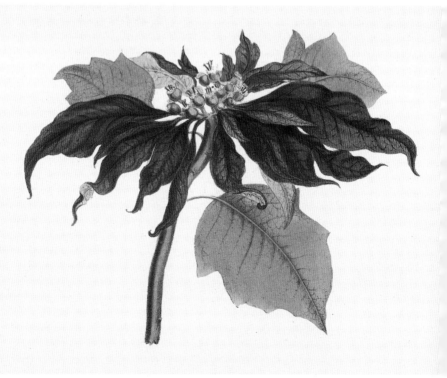

Plates 61, 62, and 63. Poinsettia (*Euphorbia pulcherrima*)

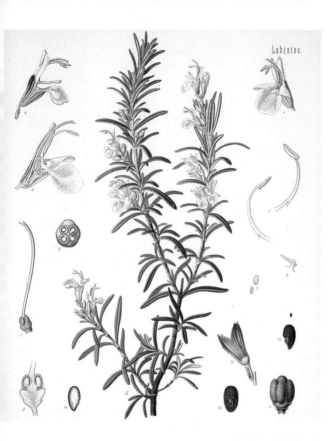

Plate 64. Rosemary
(*Rosmarinus officinalis*)

Plate 65. Star of Bethlehem
(*Ornithogalum umbellatum*)

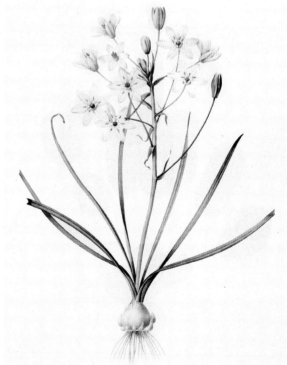

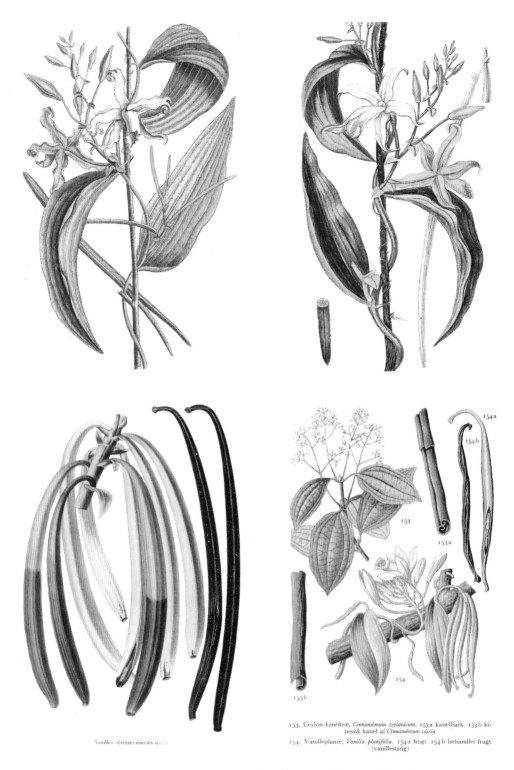

Vanilles obtenurs dans les serres

153. Ceylon-kaneltræ, *Cinnamómum zeylánicum*. 153a kanelbark. 153b kinesisk kanel af *Cinnamómum cássia*

154. Vanilleplante, *Vanilla planifólia*. 154a frugt. 154b behandlet frugt (vanillestang)

Plates 66, 67, 68, and 69. Vanilla (*Vanilla planifolia, Vanilla tahitensis, Vanilla mexicana*) and Vanilla and Cinnamon

🍃 Poinsettia-Red Cocktail for Yule

Serve this celebratory brew, hued as blood red as a poinsettia, after your Solstice rite, and make a toast in honor of the returning Sun. Be sure to use unsweetened cranberry juice, not the sweet cranberry juice cocktail sold in supermarkets.

Makes 10 servings

For the Spiced Cranberry Syrup

2 cups unsweetened, organic 100% cranberry juice (for abundance, energy, healing, and love)

1 cup organic sugar (to sweeten relationships and situations)

10 whole cardamom pods (for love and passion)

2 star anise pods (for abundance, luck, and health)

5 whole cloves (for protection from hostile or negative forces)

½ tablespoon whole allspice berries (for will, energy, money, luck, and healing)

2-inch piece of fresh organic ginger, sliced into coins (for passion, healing, luck, and energy)

Peel of 1 organic orange, cut into smallish sections (for love, luck, and prosperity and to honor the Sun)

For the Punch

1 cup Cointreau or Grand Marnier

1 cup Spiced Cranberry Syrup

6 dashes of apple-flavored bitters

Ice

1 (750-milliliter) bottle dry sparkling wine

Thin organic lemon slices, for garnish

Make the Spiced Cranberry Syrup

Combine the cranberry juice, sugar, cardamom, star anise, cloves, allspice, ginger, and orange peel in a small saucepan over medium heat. Cook, stirring

Adapted from Brian Oh's "Poinsettia Cocktail Recipe," Serious Eats (website), August 30, 2018.

continuously, until the sugar is dissolved. Let simmer for 5 minutes, then remove from the heat and let cool to room temperature.

Strain the syrup through a fine-mesh strainer or cheesecloth and set aside.

Make the Punch

Combine the Cointreau, syrup, and bitters in a large punchbowl and stir in a Sunwise (clockwise) direction.

Fill the bowl with ice, then pour in the whole bottle of sparkling wine. Stir briefly in a Sunwise direction, chanting as you stir:

> *Solstice wisdom, Solstice cheer,*
> *Solstice Spirit, welcome here!**

Ladle the punch into glasses, garnishing each with a lemon slice, and serve immediately.

---

*The chant is by Selena Fox, Pagan Priestess of Circle Sanctuary, a Nature Spirituality church.

Rosemary
(*Rosmarinus officinalis*)
·················· 🌿 ··················

There's rosemary, that's for remembrance. Pray you, love,
remember. And there is pansies, that's for thoughts.
WILLIAM SHAKESPEARE, *HAMLET* (CA. 1602)

Where rosemary flourishes, the lady rules.
TRADITIONAL BRITISH SAYING

According to lore, the Palm tree, Juniper, Willow, and Rosemary were plants that sheltered the Virgin Mary and the baby Jesus as they fled into Egypt to escape the soldiers of Herod. During the flight into Egypt, Mary is said to have spread her child's clothing on a Rosemary plant to dry, and the flowers, which had been white, turned blue and gained the sweet scent we know today. At midnight on Twelfth Night, or January 5, the eve of Epiphany, it's said, Rosemary plants burst into flower in celebration of Christmas.[167]

The ancient Romans wore crowns of fragrant Rosemary at feasts such as the Saturnalia revels, and ancient Greek scholars wore crowns of Rosemary in their hair to help them focus and memorize for exams. This is why the old Latin name for this herb was *Rosmarinus coronarius* (the Latin *coronarious* means "crown").

The Romans burned Rosemary as incense and used it to decorate and to honor the Lares or household Gods. The evergreen leaves of the plant made it a symbol of immortality and an herb of choice at funerals.

Rosemary was once a popular herb for wedding bouquets and crowns as well. As seventeenth-century poet Robert Herrick observed in his poem "The Rosemary Branch":

> *Grow for two ends, it matters not at all,*
> *Be 't for my bridal or my burial.*

Rosemary was also used to decorate the wassail bowl and to garnish the main course of the Yuletide feast, such as boar or roast beef. In German tradition, it is said to bring joy to the family when it is burned in the house on Christmas Eve.[168]

Medicinal Properties

A member of the Mint family, Rosemary is used by herbalists to ease muscle pain, strengthen memory, boost the immune and circulatory systems, and aid digestion. It is full of antioxidants and is a natural anti-inflammatory. Simmer the leaves in wine or add them to salves for rheumatism, eczema, bruises, and sores. Rosemary tea can be taken as a mouthwash for bad breath and used as a hair rinse to increase hair growth.

According to modern studies, the Greeks had it right: This herb really does improve mental concentration, performance, speed, and accuracy as well as mood. It can aid in cognitive recovery for those who have had a stroke and could help prevent brain aging.

Rosemary also has antitumor properties, especially for leukemia and breast carcinoma. It is very beneficial to the eyes and may help eye diseases such as age-related macular degeneration as it contains carnosic acid, which protects retinas from degeneration.[169]

The dosage depends on the preparation:

Tea: Steep 2 teaspoons of leaves per cup of freshly boiled water, covered, for 5 minutes or longer (as with any tea, the longer it steeps the stronger the flavor will be). Take ¼ cup four times a day. (For external use, such as a hair rinse, the tea can be stronger.)

Tincture: Take 5 to 20 drops, depending on the severity of the illness, in water or tea.[170]

> **CAUTION: Overuse and high doses of this herb can cause vomiting, spasms, coma, and pulmonary edema (fluid in the lungs). Pregnant women should avoid it as it can cause miscarriage. Anyone taking anticoagulants, ACE inhibitors, diuretics, or lithium should consult with a health provider before beginning medicinal use of Rosemary.[171]**

Magical Uses

Rosemary is said to foster love, remembrance, and fertility, making it a perfect herb for a wedding or handfasting. Twine Rosemary branches into a wedding crown and give bunches of Rosemary tied with ribbon to the guests.

Tradition holds that Rosemary grows best in a house where the woman rules, so women should carry it on their person or in a Spirit bag to gain personal power and success.

Rosemary is for all types of remembrance so students cramming for exams can add a few drops of the essential oil to their bath or wear it on their person as they study.[172]

Rosemary is an herb of purification and sanctification. Use the fresh branches to decorate the altar, and burn it as incense before a ritual. Crush the fresh leaves with your mortar and pestle and use them (or Rosemary essential oil) to anoint and purify your ritual tools.

Cast Rosemary branches onto a coffin at a funeral, and hand small bunches tied with ribbon to the mourners. Burn Rosemary to purify the home of negative forces and as an aid to meditation. Hang a bunch on the front door or on a gatepost to repel ill-intentioned intruders. Make a Rosemary wreath for the door or hang one inside the home to pull in positive solar vibes.

Burn Rosemary alone or with crushed Juniper berries in the sick room, or use it to fill a healing poppet. Use Rosemary with other purifying herbs, such as Cedar, Lavender, Mugwort, or Sage, to make a purifying smudge stick.

This herb also can be used as a substitute for Frankincense in magical work.[173]

Rosemary at Yuletide

Fragrant Rosemary is an herb of the Sun. Hang a wreath of Rosemary on the door, or incorporate it into a wreath of Pine and other evergreens. Place it on the Solstice altar and burn it during your ceremony. Make Orange and Clove pomanders, arrange them on a plate, and decorate the plate with branches of Rosemary. Use Rosemary to decorate the main dish on the Solstice table. Burn dried Rosemary with crushed dried Orange peel and crushed Cinnamon sticks to scent the home. Put some Rosemary in a pot with Apple slices, Orange Slices, Cloves, Cinnamon sticks, and a small branch of Pine. Leave it on the stove to simmer and perfume the house.

🌿 Garlic and Rosemary Cast Iron Skillet Bread

Every Kitchen Witch and Hearth Druid should have at least one cast iron pot or pan. Use yours to make this delicious and magical flatbread. The garlic and rosemary are purifying and protective for the home and your guests. For best effect, serve the bread right out of the oven. Have your fellow ritualists assist you in the kitchen for added merriment and fun.

Makes 6 servings

> 1 cup lukewarm water
>
> 1 tablespoon organic sugar
>
> 1 tablespoon active dry yeast
>
> 1¼ teaspoons sea salt or kosher salt
>
> ¼ cup plus 2 tablespoons organic cold-pressed virgin
> olive oil, plus more for drizzling on the finished bread

Adapted from Karen's "Garlic and Rosemary Skillet Bread," *The Food Charlatan* (blog), October 18, 2016.

2¼ cups organic all-purpose or bread flour, plus more as
needed
2 small cloves organic garlic, minced (for the dough)
2 cloves organic garlic, thinly sliced (for the top of the bread)
4 sprigs fresh rosemary, chopped, or 2 teaspoons dried

Combine the lukewarm water, sugar, and yeast in a large bowl and stir together with a spoon. Let sit for 5 minutes. The mixture should become bubbly and foamy. (If not, your yeast is dead and you'll need to start over with fresh yeast.)

Add ¾ teaspoon salt, ¼ cup olive oil, and the flour. Stir together with a spoon until a soft dough forms. Add the minced garlic and half of the rosemary to the dough and stir.

Turn the dough out onto a well-floured work surface and knead for 8 to 10 minutes. Add more flour as needed to prevent stickiness. While kneading, chant:

Queen of the Moon, Queen of the Sun,
Queen of the Heavens, Queen of the Stars,
Queen of the Waters, Queen of the Earth,
We celebrate the Sun's rebirth!

Grease a large bowl. Scrape the dough into the bowl, form it into a ball, and turn it in the bowl to coat it with oil. Cover the bowl with plastic wrap and let the dough rise for 45 minutes.

Coat a 10-inch cast iron skillet with 1 tablespoon of olive oil.

Take the plastic wrap off the bowl with the dough; save it for the second rising. Punch down the dough, then transfer it to the cast iron skillet, pressing it into the bottom of the pan.

Use a sharp knife to deeply score the top of the dough with a solar cross or sun-wheel pattern. Brush the top with the remaining 1 tablespoon of olive oil. Sprinkle with sliced garlic, the rest of the rosemary, and the remaining ½ teaspoon salt. Cover loosely with plastic wrap and let rise another 20 minutes.

Meanwhile, preheat the oven to 400°F.

Bake the bread for 20 to 25 minutes, until the top is light golden brown all over. Remove from the oven. Take the bread out the skillet right away and let cool briefly on a wire rack.

Drizzle with olive oil, slice into wedges, and serve hot!

Star of Bethlehem
(*Ornithogalum umbellatum*)
......................🌿......................

*When the Star of Bethlehem flowers surround your house,
it is a powerful sign. You are being strongly protected and
purified. Some people see these flowers as a sign of hope.*
BRENDA MARIE FLUHARTY, "SPIRITUAL PROTECTION:
THE STAR OF BETHLEHEM FLOWERS"

A member of the Hyacinthaceae (winter lily) family, Star of Bethlehem is native to Europe, North Africa, and western Asia but widely naturalized in the United States. It gets its name from its supposed resemblance to the supernova that heralded Jesus's birth (never mind that it blooms in April or May!).

Its white petals, according to a French legend, sprang into being when the biblical Star of Bethlehem appeared. To Mary's amazement, the white flowers emerged from the dried weeds and hay of the manger and formed a crown upon the head of the newborn Jesus.[174]

Another legend holds that the star that appeared in the sky over Bethlehem to guide the Wise Astrologers was too beautiful to banish from the universe after they had found Jesus, so the star burst into thousands of pieces and descended to Earth. There, it became the white flower we know today.[175]

A hardy perennial, Star of Bethlehem resurrects itself year after year, further echoing the legend of the risen Christ.

Medicinal Properties
Star of Bethlehem has traditionally been used to relieve coughs, strengthen the heart, improve memory, relieve acute chronic diarrhea, expel intestinal parasites, decrease lung congestion, and decrease water retention in the legs. It treats digestive disturbances such as gas, improves liver and kidney function, soothes bladder inflammation, improves osteoporosis, and relieves the pain of arthritis and rheumatism. The plant acts similarly to digoxin and can be used to treat high blood pressure and dizziness.

Externally, the tea is added to the bath or used as a wash for irritated skin, eczema, dermatitis, bruising, hematoma, and wounds.

The leaves should be used as medicine in the spring and the bulbs in the fall. Both can be chopped and eaten in salads (they taste like Garlic) and used to flavor meats, egg dishes, and breads.

For stomach problems and for a winter immune boost, steep the chopped flowers in wine for 24 hours, strain, and take small sips every few hours.

Make a summer Sun tincture by placing the chopped flowers in alcohol. Leave the jar in the Sun for 3 weeks, then strain. Take 20 drops three times a day for 2 weeks in water, tea, or soup.[176]

> **CAUTION: Use Star of Bethlehem only with expert supervision, as this herb contains powerful cardiac glycosides that can lead to irregular heartbeat and even death. Pregnant and breastfeeding women should avoid it altogether. Do not use it in combination with antibiotics, as they can make the plant's constituents more bioavailable to your body and exacerbate reactions to the herb. Do not take it in combination with digoxin, as it has similar properties. Also do not take it with quinine, stimulant laxatives, or diuretics.[177]**
>
> **The bulbs and foliage contain toxic alkaloids. Grow them in areas that won't tempt your dog, cat, or livestock, especially horses, to nibble the leaves.[178]**

Star of Bethlehem is one of the original thirty-eight Bach Flower remedies. Dr. Edward Bach described its uses as follows:

> For those in great distress under conditions which for a time produce great unhappiness. The shock of serious news, the loss of some one dear, the fright following an accident, and such like. For those who for a time refuse to be consoled this remedy brings comfort.[179]

Dr. Bach combined Star of Bethlehem flower essence (for shock) with the flower essences of Rock Rose (for terror), Impatiens (for frustration and irritability), Cherry Plum (for fear), and Clematis (for drowsiness and lightheadedness) to make an all-purpose emergency remedy he named Rescue Remedy.

I have meditated with Star of Bethlehem to understand how Bach came to his conclusions about it. In my garden at least, the appearance of the flowers means the time of frost and snow are fully over, heralding a recovery from the frozen grip of deadly winter.

Flower essences are made by placing the flowers in a crystal bowl and barely covering them with water. They are left exposed to the Sun for 4 hours on a cloudless day. Then the water is strained and alcohol (40 percent alcohol by volume), such as fruit brandy, is added as a preservative. This is not a Sun tea; it is a light potentiation.

Magical Uses

Grow the bulbs inside on a sunny windowsill in winter, or bring the cut flowers into the home in the spring, for spiritual protection and to support a sense of hope.

The white flowers bestow a sense of balance, cleansing, harmony, purity, and serenity. The blue flowers enhance trust, respect, and honesty. The orange and yellow flowers bring optimism, happiness, and joy. The purple flowers bequeath beauty, mastery, and a key to the mysteries.[180]

Star of Bethlehem at Yuletide

Place the white or yellow flowers on the altar in honor of the return of our nearest star, the Sun. Fill your home with the flowers, and gift the bulbs to friends to be grown on winter windowsills.

> *Ornithogalon has a tender stalk—thin, whitish, about two feet high—with three or four tender slips growing together on the top from which come the flowers, which outwardly seem the colour of herbs but opened they are similar to milk. Between them is a little head . . . that is baked together with bread. . . . The root is bulbous and is eaten both raw and boiled.*
> DIOSCORIDES, *DE MATERIA MEDICA* (CA. 50–70 CE), TRANS. T. A. OSBALDESTON AND R. P. A. WOOD

Fried Star of Bethlehem

There are wildly conflicting reports about the toxicity or edibility of this plant. *The ancients ate it raw or cooked, according to Dioscorides, and it does feature in some indigenous cuisines. For example, people in Turkey eat the roots, cleaning them carefully, boiling them until soft, squeezing out the liquid, and sautéing them with onions and scrambled eggs.*[181] *The Greeks use the greens in pies.*[182] *The roots and greens are sometimes chopped and made into fritters, coated in egg and breadcrumb mixtures and fried, or added to breads.*

It would seem that the safest way to use the bulbs and greens is in cooked dishes, but foragers I know have eaten the fresh bulbs with no ill results. As with all wild foods, please test a bit first and see how it affects you. And do not use commercially cultivated bulbs as food. Use only organically grown bulbs from nature or from your own (organic) garden!

Do not feed the root, leaves, or flowers to a dog or cat. It will make them very sick. It is also toxic to horses.

  2 servings

> 250 grams star of Bethlehem bulbs, chopped
> 2 teaspoons salt
> 2 free-range organic eggs
> 1 cup organic vegetable oil

Bring enough water to cover the star of Bethlehem to a boil. Add the star of Bethlehem and boil for 3 minutes and drain thoroughly.

Return the star of Bethlehem to the pot, add in the salt, and mix until spread evenly.

Heat the oil in a pan.

Beat the eggs in a separate bowl and coat the star of Bethlehem.

Fry both sides of the star of Bethlehem to desired crispness.

Adapted from Sevinç Karabak's "Fried Star of Bethlehem," Biodiversity for Food and Nutrution (website), accessed 3/20/2023.

Vanilla
(*Vanilla planifolia, Vanilla tahitensis*)
.... 🌿 ....

The word comes from Greek mythology. Orchis was the son of a satyr and a nymph. During a feast to celebrate Bacchus, Orchis drank too much wine and tried to force his attentions on a priestess. Bacchus was very displeased, and reacted by having Orchis torn to pieces. The pieces were scattered far and wide, and wherever one landed, an orchid grew.

LISA KLEYPAS, *COLD-HEARTED RAKE* (2015)

An aphrodisiac since antiquity, Vanilla bean is the second-most expensive spice in the world, after Saffron (*Crocus sativus*). The beans are the edible fruits of a tropical orchid. The Olmec people on the Gulf Coast of present-day Mexico were probably the first to use Vanilla as a food flavoring. At the time, wild Vanilla was already being used as a fragrance in temples, and the flowers were placed in amulets for protection from the evil eye.[183]

Vanilla orchids were eventually domesticated by the pre-Colombian Totonac people of Mexico. According to their lore, the Vanilla orchid rose from the blood of the divine princess Tzacopontziza (Morning Star), who had been forbidden to marry by her father. She then dedicated her life to Tonoacayohua, the Goddess of plants and the harvest. As fate would have it, the princess encountered a young mortal man and fell in love. The two lovers fled into the forest but were captured by angry priests of the Goddess and beheaded. Each drop of blood that fell from the princess was transformed into a Vanilla orchid, and each drop of blood that fell from her lover became a bush upon which the orchids twined.

When the Totonac people were eventually conquered by the Aztecs, their conquerors began using Vanilla to flavor their *cacahuatl*, a drink made from water, honey, ground corn, and cocoa. The Aztecs thought of Vanilla as an aphrodisiac and required the Totonac people to pay their taxes in the form of Vanilla beans.

In the sixteenth century, Hernán Cortés and the Spanish conquistadores defeated the Aztecs and sent the first Vanilla beans to Europe. Hugh Morgan, apothecary to England's Queen Elizabeth, had the idea to use the flavor in a range of products, including perfumes, tobacco, and alcohol. Vanilla consumption took off in the United States thanks to Thomas Jefferson, who added it to his ice cream (see the recipe below).[184]

For three hundred years, Vanilla beans were produced exclusively in their native Mexico. The orchids were transported to other tropical regions and planted, but without their native pollinators, none produced fruit until Edmond Albius, a twelve-year-old boy enslaved on the island of Réunion, discovered that the plants could be successfully hand-pollinated using a blade of grass. Now four regions produce most of the world's Vanilla, each with a slightly different taste: Indonesia, Madagascar, Mexico, and Tahiti.[185]

Medicinal Properties

Vanilla is rich in antioxidants and is used to relieve intestinal gas and fever, lower cholesterol, and lower stress, which can speed healing. It is also used as an aphrodisiac to increase sexual desire.[186]

Vanilla is rich in magnesium and potassium, which are vital for kidney, heart, muscle, and nerve function. One of its constituents, vanillin, has antidepressant effects comparable to those of a common antidepressant medication known as fluoxetine (Prozac). (But, of course, do not take yourself off Prozac without a doctor's supervision.)

Vanillin and two other constituents, ethyl vanillin and vanillic acid, have antibacterial activity that combats *Cronobacter* species, a group of bacteria that can cause severe and sometimes fatal infections in infants, the elderly, and people with compromised immune systems.[187]

Drinking Vanilla herbal tea soothes gut inflammation and helps with digestive problems such as cramping, stomachache, and diarrhea. Steep about ½ tsp. real Vanilla bean pods—scraped and cut up—per cup of water for 15 minutes and strain. Take a total of 1 cup of this tea per day in 1/4 cup amounts in between meals.

If you have a cough, cold, or respiratory infection, drink pure Vanilla extract mixed with a little warm water to help coat the throat and provide an anesthetic effect. Its antibacterial properties help reduce inflammation and irritation. Vanilla's natural appetite-suppressing qualities can also help in a weight loss program; try taking the extract in hot water or tea. The dosage for Vanilla extract as medicinal remedy is 1 teaspoon per day, in hot water or tea.

Externally, Vanilla essential oil strengthens the hair and stimulates blood flow in the scalp, leading to increased hair growth.[188] You can also rub the extract into the scalp and rinse with water and a little more extract for the same effect. Apply the extract diluted in water to acne, burns, wounds, and cuts. Vanilla relieves pain and inflammation and fights infection.

> **CAUTION: Skin contact and excessive external use can cause irritation and swelling (inflammation) in some individuals. It might also cause headache and sleep problems (insomnia). While pregnant and breastfeeding women can safely enjoy Vanilla as a food flavoring, they should avoid it as a medicine until more is known of its effects.**

Magical Uses

In addition to the love lore of Vanilla and the Totonac people noted above, Vanilla is also sacred to Aphrodite/Venus, making it an obvious choice for love spells. At the same time, its calming qualities and antibacterial properties suggest it as a good herb for healing rites and potions.

To draw in love, place a Vanilla bean into a jar with some sugar and a piece of rose quartz. As you hold the jar between your hands, visualize yourself as loved, whether by a friend, a parent, a sibling, a lover, or any other category of person. Place the jar in a safe place and hold it when you feel the need for more love in your life. Add the sugar to warm tea when you need comfort.[189]

Vanilla is also an herb of protection; wear the bean or a piece of a bean in a Spirit bag under your clothing to ward off jealousy and ill intentions.

Add Vanilla essential oil or extract to your bath to attract love.

Vanilla at Yuletide

Prepare a Yule or Christmas recipe containing Vanilla: eggnog, a cake, cookies, pudding, hot chocolate, candies, or whatever you prefer. The possibilities are endless. As you cook, visualize the spirit of this beautiful plant working with you to create joy and affection in your family and world. If your Yule gathering could use a bit of extra calming and tenderness, consider spraying water with a bit of Vanilla extract added all through the house.

🌶 Thomas Jefferson's Vanilla Ice Cream

Thomas Jefferson's original recipe for making vanilla ice cream is now housed in the Library of Congress. You can make it a Yuletide treat by pouring on hot chocolate syrup and a sprinkle of chopped candied ginger. It's a perfect dessert for your Solstice soiree, with vanilla for eternal love, chocolate for community bonding, and ginger for passion.

Makes 2¼ quarts

> 2 quarts organic heavy whipping cream
> 1 cup organic sugar
> 1 vanilla bean*
> 6 free-range organic egg yolks

Combine the cream and sugar in a large pan. Split the vanilla bean in half lengthwise. Using a sharp knife, scrape the seeds into the pan and then drop in the bean.

Put the egg yolks in a small bowl. Get out a large bowl, and prepare a pan of ice water big enough to hold the large bowl.

Heat the cream mixture over medium heat until bubbles form around the sides of pan, whisking Sunwise (clockwise) all the while to dissolve the sugar. As you stir, chant:

Adapted from Taste of Home's "Thomas Jefferson's Vanilla Ice Cream," Taste of Home (website), accessed December 7, 2021.

---

*If you don't have a real vanilla bean, substitute 1 tablespoon vanilla extract. Stir the extract into the cream mixture after the ice-water bath.

Gathered here in mystery,
Gathered in one strong body,
Gathered here in our power,
Spirit (or health, love, Solstice,
abundance, etc.) drawing near.

Ladle a small portion of the hot cream mixture into the egg yolks to temper them. Then pour the yolk mixture into the pan, whisking constantly to prevent curdling. (Keep chanting!)

Cook over low heat, stirring constantly, until the mixture is just thick enough to coat a metal spoon and the temperature reaches 160°F. Do not allow it to boil.

When the mixture reaches the right temperature, immediately transfer it to the large bowl you got out earlier. Place the bowl in the pan of ice water. Stir gently and occasionally for 2 minutes. (Keep chanting!)

Remove and discard the vanilla bean. Press waxed paper onto the surface of the custard and refrigerate for several hours or overnight. (If there is snow outside, why not leave it out under the winter sky?)

Fill the cylinder of an ice cream freezer two-thirds full with the custard, and freeze according to the manufacturer's directions. Refrigerate the remaining mixture until you are ready to freeze it.

When it's ready, transfer the ice cream to a freezer container; freeze for 4 to 6 hours, until firm.

NOTES

AN INTRODUCTION TO
YULE AND HERBAL MAGIC

1. "The Red Road," Spirit Horse Nation (website), accessed February 28, 2020; "Red: Colors in Polish Folklore (Part 1)," *Lamus Dworski* (blog), June 15, 2019.

2. Ivan F. Star Comes Out, "Ivan Star: Sharing Lakota Perspectives and Meanings of Colors," *Native Sun News* (online), December 23, 2014.

3. "White: Colors in Polish Folklore (Part 2)," *Lamus Dworski* (blog), June 17, 2019.

4. Gerry Bowler, *The World Encyclopedia of Christmas* (Toronto: McClelland and Stewart, 2000), 148.

THE GIFT BRINGERS, SPIRITS,
AND MYSTICAL FIGURES OF WINTER

1. Gerry Bowler, *The World Encyclopedia of Christmas* (Toronto: McClelland and Stewart, 2000), 155–56.

2. Charlotte McDonald-Gibson, "The Fight Over 'Black Pete' Brings a Reckoning on Racial Equality in the Netherlands," Time (website), November 14, 2020.

3. "Knecht Ruprecht," *Encyclopedia of Christmas and New Year's Celebrations,* 2nd ed. (online; Omnigraphics, Inc., 2003), accessed February 28, 2021.

4. Bowler, *The World Encyclopedia of Christmas,* 18, 21–22, 128, 193.

5. "Tomte and Santa," Swedishfood.com (website), accessed March 20, 2021; "A Little Background on the Scandinavian Julenisse and Christmas Pixie," Fjorn (website), accessed March 20, 2021.

6. Bowler, *World Encyclopedia of Christmas,* 15, 208.

7. "The Ladies of Christmas," Writing in the Margins (website), accessed February 22, 2021.

8. "Goddess Abundantia," General Spirituality Wiki (website), accessed February 27, 2021.

9. Bowler, *World Encyclopedia of Christmas,* 19.

10. Bowler, *World Encyclopedia of Christmas,* 138, 149.

11. Bowler, *World Encyclopedia of Christmas,* 22, 104.

12. Bowler, *World Encyclopedia of Christmas,* 135.

13. "Star Symbolism and Christmas Gift-Bringers from Polish Folklore," *Lamus Dworski* (blog), December 17, 2016.

14. Bowler, *World Encyclopedia of Christmas,* 91.

15. "Christmas in France: Twelve Traditions That Make a French Christmas," The Local (website), December 13, 2018; Helen Parkinson, "4 Legendary Christmas Characters in France and Where to Find Them," Complete France (website), accessed February 22, 2021.

16. Bowler, *World Encyclopedia of Christmas,* 220.

17. Bowler, *World Encyclopedia of Christmas,* 46.

18. Regína Hrönn Ragnarsdóttir, "Grýla and Leppalúði—the Parents of the Icelandic Yule Lads," Guide to Iceland (website), accessed March 14, 2021.

19. Susan, "Kallikantzaroi—Greek Christmas Goblins—Greek Christmas Customs & Traditions," Greeker Than the Greeks (website), accessed March 22, 2021; Dolores Reyes Pergioudakis, "Greek Christmas Elves," *Pleasanton Express* (online), December 23, 2014; Bowler, *World Encyclopedia of Christmas,* 97.

20. Bowler, *World Encyclopedia of Christmas,* 246.

21. Zanna Jezek, "The Tradition of Svatý Mikuláš," Très Bohèmes (website), December 5, 2016.

22. Bowler, *World Encyclopedia of Christmas,* 251.

23. Bowler, *World Encyclopedia of Christmas,* 248.

THE ANIMALS AT YULE

1. Gerry Bowler, *The World Encyclopedia of Christmas* (Toronto: McClelland and Stewart, 2000), 9–10.

2. Bowler, *World Encyclopedia of Christmas,* 108.

3. Ben Jones, "Introduction to Hoodening," Hoodening.org (website), accessed February 28, 2021.

4. "Rodanthe Old Christmas Is Older Than Rodanthe," *Outer Banks Blue* (blog), December 5, 2017.

5. A. W. Moore, *Folklore of the Isle of Man* (London: Brown & Son, 1891), 102.

6. E. C. Cawte, *Ritual Animal Disguise: A Historical and Geographical Study of Animal Disguise in the British Isles* (Cambridge and Totowa: D. S. Brewer Ltd. and Rowman and Littlefield for the Folklore Society, 1978), 144, 147.

7. Saryn Chorney, "Who Runs the Sleigh? Girls! Science Says Santa's Reindeer Are Actually All Female," People (website), accessed March 2, 2021.

8. Douglas Main, "8 Ways Magic Mushrooms Explain Santa Story," LiveScience.com (website), accessed March 2, 2021.

9. Bowler, *World Encyclopedia of Christmas,* 191.

10. Alexei Kondratiev, *The Apple Branch* (Cork: Collins Press, 1998), 128.

11. R. I. Best, *Prognostications from the Raven and the Wren* (Eriu, 1916).

RITUALS AND RITES OF SOLSTICE, YULE, AND CHRISTMAS

1. Philip Chrysopoulos, "Podariko: Why Greeks Select Who Sets Foot First in the House on New Year," Greek Reporter (website), December 31, 2022.

2. Gerry Bowler, *The World Encyclopedia of Christmas* (Toronto: McClelland and Stewart, 2000), 31, 844, 105.

3. Bowler, *World Encyclopedia of Christmas,* 54.

4. Ronald Hutton, *Stations of the Sun: A History of the Ritual Year in Britain* (OUP Oxford, 2001), 95.

5. Ben Cousins, "What Is Belsnickeling? Unpacking a Holiday Tradition among 'Most Nova Scotians,'" CTV News (website), November 22, 2018.

6. Jacob Brown, *Brown's Miscellaneous Writings* (Cumberland, Maryland: J. J. Miller, 1896), 41.

7. Dale M. Brumfield, "Belsnickeling and Shanghaiing: Forgotten County Traditions," News Leader, January 15, 2017.

8. Arthur Machen, "Dog and Duck," in *Dog and Duck* (Jonathan Cape, 1924).

9. Pixyled Publications, "Custom Demised: Calennig on New Year's Day," *Traditional Ceremonies and Customs* (blog), January 31, 2016.

10. Christian Langenegger, "Alter Silvester Is a Swiss Tradition That Lives On," *Newly Swissed* (blog), January 14, 2013.

11. William D. Crump, *Encyclopedia of New Year's Holidays Worldwide* (North Carolina and London: McFarland & Company, 2008), 88.

12. Tim Sandles, "Ashen Faggot," Legendary Dartmoor (website), accessed February 7, 2021.

13. Bowler, *World Encyclopedia of Christmas,* 254–55.

14. Bowler, *World Encyclopedia of Christmas,* 15–16, 130.

15. "Ashen Faggot," *Wikipedia* (website), accessed February 7, 2021.

16. "The Burning of the Clavie," Burghead.com (website), accessed February 6, 2021; "Why Do We Celebrate the Burning of the Clavie?" The Scottish Hampers (website), accessed February 6, 2021.

17. Carolin Schratt, "The Magic of the Rauhnächte," *Kleinwalsertal* (blog), December 12, 2013.

18. James Orchard Halliwell, Esq., *A Catalogue of Chap-Books, Garlands and Popular Histories,* private collection, from the British Museum, London, 1849.

19. Vlada Koroleva, "Russian Christmas," Just Russian (website/blog), accessed May 2, 2023.

20. Irina Bekreniova, "St. Andrew's Day in Ukraine: Vechornytsy," Into English (website), accessed April 4, 2021.

21. "St Andrew's Day Tales and Traditions," Scotland.org (website), accessed April 4, 2021.

22. Bowler, *World Encyclopedia of Christmas,* 236, 244.

23. "Christmas Kutia. What Is Kutya: History, Types and Secrets of Cooking," Geotoriya (website), accessed April 5, 2021.

24. Bowler, *World Encyclopedia of Christmas,* 18.

25. Robert Herrick, "Ceremony Upon Candlemas Eve," in *Works of Robert Herrrick,* vol. 2, ed. Alfred Pollard (London: Lawrence and Bullen, 1891).

26. Bowler, *World Encyclopedia of Christmas,* 35, 241.

CHRISTMAS TRADITIONS AND RECIPES
FROM AROUND THE WORLD

1. Gerry Bowler, *The World Encyclopedia of Christmas* (Toronto: McClelland and Stewart, 2000), 183.

2. "Some French Christmas Traditions," Alpine French School (website), accessed January 17, 2021.

3. Sébastien Nantel, "5 Days of French-Canadian Christmas Traditions—Le Réveillon," *Painted Puffin* (blog), December 14, 2011.

4. "Christmas Customs in Greece," Greeka (website), December 20, 2013.

5. "How Italians Do Christmas: The Foods You'll Find on Every Table," Devour Rome (website), accessed January 6, 2021.

6. Bowler, *World Encyclopedia of Christmas,* 133.

7. "Examples of a Podłaźniczka," *Lamus Dworski* (blog), accessed April 15, 2021.

8. "Polish Christmas Traditions: How Do We Celebrate Christmas in Poland?" Travel Poland (website), accessed January 23, 2021.

9. Bowler, *World Encyclopedia of Christmas,* 178.

10. James Cooper, "Christmas in Russia," whychristmas.com (website), accessed January 15, 2021.

11. David Pope, "7 Spanish Christmas Traditions to Celebrate This Year," Spanish Sabores (website), accessed January 25, 2021.

12. Esme Fox, "The Top 10 Spanish Traditional Christmas Foods," Culture Trip (website), accessed January 25, 2021.

13. Jean Williams, "Jul: Scandinavian Yuletide," *Deseret News* (online), December 14, 1993.

14. "Christmas in Sweden," whychristmas.com (website), accessed January 27, 2021.

15. "Christmas in Sweden," whychristmas.com (website), accessed January 27, 2021.

16. "Swiss Christmas Traditions," Alpenwild (website), accessed January 28, 2021.

17. "Swiss Christmas Foods," Alpenwild (website), accessed January 28, 2021.

18. Ayngelina Brogan, "A Guide to Christmas in Venezuela," Tripsavvy (website), January 20, 2020.

19. "Christmas in Venezuela," TheHolidaySpot (website), February 1, 2021.

20. Annette McDermott, "Venezuelan Christmas Traditions: From Gifts to Music," Love to Know (website), accessed January 28, 2023.

21. Ben Johnson, "Welsh Christmas Traditions," Historic UK (website), accessed January 29, 2021.

WASSAILING AND
OTHER YULETIDE LIBATIONS

1. "Wassail," Central Lakes Clinic (website), December 9, 2020.

2. Pixyled Publications, "Custom Demised: The Vessel or Wassail Cup," *Traditional Ceremonies and Customs* (blog), December 31, 2015.

3. "The Epiphany," in *Christmas in Ritual & Tradition* (online book, n.d.), 345.

4. "Wassail Toast," from the Dunton Wassail 2015 flyer of the Dunton Folk, available online.

5. Gerry Bowler, *The World Encyclopedia of Christmas* (Toronto: McClelland and Stewart, 2000), 242–43.

6. Leslie Anneliese, "Wassailing, Old Tradition Made New," *Radiant Nursing* (blog), accessed February 28, 2021.

7. Ross Dennis, as quoted by Sean Murphy in "Traditional Scottish Recipe: The Hot Toddy," The Scotsman (website), February 19, 2016.

8. "Persephone, Queen of the Underworld," Greeka (website), accessed May 26, 2021.

PART TWO:
MAGICAL AND MEDICINAL HERBS OF WINTER

1. Lei Zhang and Bal L. Lokeshwar, "Medicinal Properties of the Jamaican Pepper Plant *Pimenta dioica* and Allspice," *Current Drug Targets* 13, no. 14 (2012).

2. Cathy Wong, "The Benefits of Allspice," VeryWellHealth (website), accessed May 18, 2021.

3. "Allspice," RxList (website), accessed May 18, 2021.

4. "The Structure of the Menorah," Construction of the Menorah and the Bible (website), accessed May 19, 2021.

5. M. Guasch-Ferré, X. Liu, V. S. Malik, et al., "Nut Consumption and Risk of Cardiovascular Disease," *Journal of the American College of Cardiology* 70, no. 20 (2017): 2519–32.

6. "Almonds," Nutrition Source (website) of the Harvard T. H. Chan School of Public Health, accessed May 20, 2021.

7. "Sweet Almond—Uses, Side Effects, and More," WebMD (website), accessed May 21, 2021.

8. "Magical Properties of Almonds," on the Tumblr blog of iridescent-witch-life, July 24, 2020.

9. Maria Short et al., "How to Add Color to Marzipan," wikiHow (website), accessed May 20, 2021.

10. M. B. Henry, "Why Apples? A Tale of Eden and Christmas Trees," M. B. Henry: Following the Path to the Past (website), November 29, 2018.

11. P. Knekt, S. Isotupa, H. Rissanen, et al., "Quercetin Intake and the Incidence of Cerebrovascular Disease," *European Journal of Clinical Nutrition* 54 (2000): 415–17.

12. M. P. McRae, "Dietary Fiber Is Beneficial for the Prevention of Cardiovascular Disease: An Umbrella Review of Meta-analyses," *Journal of Chiropractic Medicine* 16, no. 4 (2017): 289–99.

13. G. Ravn-Haren, L. O. Dragsted, T. Buch-Andersen, et al. "Intake of Whole Apples or Clear Apple Juice Has Contrasting Effects on Plasma Lipids in Healthy Volunteers," *European Journal of Nutrition* 52 (2013): 1875–89.

14. R. Fabiani, L. Minelli, and P. Rosignoli, "Apple Intake and Cancer Risk: A Systematic Review and Meta-analysis of Observational Studies," *Public Health Nutrition* 19, no. 14 (2016): 2603–17.

15. Richard Whelan, "Bayberry," Herbs from A–Z (website), accessed May 29, 2021.

16. John Lust, *The Herb Book* (New York: Bantam, 1974), 391.

17. Michelle Gruben, "Magickal Properties of Bayberry," Grove and Grotto (website), December 16, 2016.

18. Joybilee Farm, "DIY Bayberry Candle from Foraged Berries," Joybilee Farm (website), accessed May 29, 2021.

19. S. Rastogi, M. M. Pandey, and A. Kumar Singh Rawat, "Medicinal Plants of the Genus Betula—Traditional Uses and a Phytochemical-Pharmacological Review," *Journal of Ethnopharmacology* 159 (2015): 62–83, doi:10.1016/j.jep.2014.11.010.

20. Lust, *The Herb Book,* 117–18.

21. "Birch," WebMD (website), accessed May 30, 2021.

22. Barbara Drake Boehm and Alexandra Suda, "What Is Boxwood?" AGO: The Boxwood Project, accessed May 30, 2021.

23. Thor Sturluson, "Boxwood—Health Benefits and Side Effects," Herbal Resource (website), accessed May 30, 2021.

24. Richard Folkard, *Plant Lore, Legends, and Lyrics* (London: Sampson Low, Marston, Searle, and Rivington, 1884), 256.

25. "What Useful Properties Does Boxwood Have?" Yellow Bread (website), accessed May 30, 2021.

26. "The History of Chocolate," HowStuffWorks.com (website), November 18, 2007.

27. Chris Kilham, "Cocoa, the Health Miracle," Medicine Hunter (website), accessed June 2, 2021.

28. "Cocoa," MedicineNet (website), accessed June 2, 2021.

29. "Cocoa," RxList (website), accessed June 2, 2021.

30. Belle Awen, "Myths and Legends about Herbs and Spices," Elementress Botanicals (website), March 27, 2019.

31. Peggy Trowbridge Filippone, "Origin and Historical Uses of Cinnamon," The Spruce Eats (website), accessed June 2, 2021.

32. P. Ranasinghe, S. Pigera, G. S. Premakumara, et al., "Medicinal Properties of 'True' Cinnamon (*Cinnamomum zeylanicum*): A Systematic Review," *BMC Complementary and Alternative Medicine* 13 (2013): 275.

33. "Can Taking Cinnamon Supplements Lower Your Blood Sugar?" Diabetes & Endocrinology subsection, healthessentials section, Clevland Clinic website, December 23, 2020.

34. Linda Lum, "Exploring Cloves: The Christmas Spice Adds a Touch of Heat to Every Meal," Delishably (website), November 24, 2022.

35. Meenakshi Nagdeve, "10 Surprising Health Benefits of Cloves," Organic Facts (website), accessed June 12, 2021.

36. "Clove—Overview, Uses, Side Effects," WebMD (website), accessed June 12, 2021.

37. Alethea Cho, "The Magical History of Pomanders," Medium (website), December 18, 2019.

38. Rebecca Andersson, "How to Make Pomanders with Oranges and Cloves," Azure (website), December 17, 2015.

39. Nantucket Conservation Foundation, "Cranberries," accessed June 17, 2021.

40. Charles V. Mathis, "The Cranberry: Ruby of the Barrens," *New York Times* (online), October 21, 1973.

41. Nantucket Conservation Foundation, "Cranberries," accessed June 17, 2021.

42. "4 Myths about Cranberry and Urinary Tract Health," Theralogix *Balanced Living Blog* (blog), accessed June 17, 2021.

43. "Cranberry—Dosing," WebMD (website), accessed June 18, 2021.

44. "Health Benefits of Cranberries," WebMD (website), November 29, 2022.

45. Sura Jeselsohn, "Frankincense Is Essential to Christmas Story, but What Is It?" *Riverdale Press* (online), December 23, 2018.

46. Martin Hesp, "The Christmas Story That Is Frankincense," Martin Hesp Food and Travel (website), accessed June 23, 2021.

47. Biblical Archaeology Society staff, "Why Did the Magi Bring Gold, Frankincense and Myrrh? Medicinal Uses of Frankincense May Help Explain the Gifts of the Magi," Biblical Archaeology Society Bible History Daily (website), December 20, 2022.

48. A. R. Al-Yasiry and B. Kiczorowska, "Frankincense—Therapeutic Properties," *Advances in Hygiene and Experimental Medicine* 70 (2016): 380–91, doi:10.5604/17322693.1200553.

49. Aaron Moncivaiz, "Boswellia (Indian Frankincense)," Healthline (website), accessed June 25, 2021.

50. Cathy Wong, "The Health Benefits of Frankincense Essential Oil," Verywell Health (website), accessed June 25, 2021.

51. Lust, *The Herb Book,* 288–89.

52. Cathy Wong, "The Health Benefits of Myrrh Essential Oil," Verywell Health (website), accessed June 25, 2021.

53. "Magical Uses of Frankincense and Myrrh," Original Botanica (website), accessed June 25, 2021.

54. Tori Avey, "The History of Gingerbread," *The History Kitchen* (blog) on PBS, December 20, 2013.

55. Armando Gonzalez Stuart, "Herbal Safety, Ginger," UTEP (website), accessed June 28, 2021.

56. LaQuinta McCall, "Magickal Uses for Ginger," *Real Hoodoo* (blog) on Tumblr, April 8, 2018.

57. Maya Corrigan, "The Surprisingly Dark History of Gingerbread," CrimeReads (website), accessed June 27, 2021.

58. Patricia Kasten, "Flowers for the Queen," *The Compass* (online), December 19, 2019.

59. SaVanna Shoemaker, "9 Impressive Health Benefits of Hawthorn Berry," Healthline (website), accessed July 1, 2021.

60. Mahalia Freed, "Hawthorn: Heart Healing from Physical to Spiritual," Traditional Roots Institute (website), accessed July 1, 2021.

61. "Hawthorn Berries Benefits," Indigo Herbs (website), accessed July 1, 2021.

62. "Hawthorn," National Center for Complementary and Integrative Health (website), accessed July 1, 2021.

63. Andrew Gaumond, "Ultimate Guide to Hibiscus Flower Meaning & Symbolism: Everything You Need to Know about Hibiscus Flower Meaning, Symbolism, History, Origins and Cultural Significance," Petal Republic (website), accessed July 2, 2021.

64. Kristin M. Stanton, "Hibiscus Flower Meanings & Symbolism + Hibiscus Planting, Care & Uses," UniGuide (website), accessed July 2, 2021.

65. "Hibiscus," Kaiser Permanente (website), accessed July 2, 2021.

66. Rena Goldman, "All You Need to Know about Hibiscus," Healthline (website), accessed July 2, 2021.

67. "Holly Mythology and Folklore," Trees for Life (website), accessed July 4, 2021.

68. Patricia L. Crown, Thomas E. Emerson, Jiyan Gu, W. Jeffrey Hurst, Timothy R. Pauketat, and Timothy Ward, "Ritual Black Drink Consumption at Cahokia," *Proceedings of the National Academy of Sciences* 109, no. 35 (August 6, 2012): 13944–49.

69. Lust, *The Herb Book,* 227.

70. Lust, *The Herb Book,* 227–29.

71. Green Deane, "Hollies: Caffein & Antioxidants," Eat the Weeds and Other Things Too (website), accessed July 26, 2021.

72. Chaeremon of Alexandria, as quoted in Porphyry, *De Abstinentia,* IV, 6.9.

73. *The Herb Companion* staff, "Herb to Know: Hyssop," *Mother Earth Living* (online), accessed July 27, 2021.

74. Adrienne Dellwo, "Health Benefits of Hyssop," Verywell Health (website), accessed July 28, 2021.

75. S. Zielinska and A. Matkowski, "Phytochemistry and Bioactivity of Aromatic and Medicinal Plants from the Genus Agastache (Lamiaceae)," *Phytochemistry Reviews* 13 (2014): 391–416, doi:10.1007 %2Fs11101-014-9349-1.

76. B. Javadi, A. Sahebkar, and A. Emami, "Medicinal Plants for the Treatment of Asthma: A Traditional Persian Medicine Perspective," *Current Pharmaceutical Design* 23, no. 11 (2017): 1623–32, doi:10.217 4/1381612822666161021143332.

77. M. S. Shon, Y. Lee, J. H. Song, et al., "Anti-aging Potential of Extracts Prepared from Fruits and Medicinal Herbs Cultivated in the Gyeongnam Area of Korea," *Preventive Nutrition and Food Science* 19, no. 3 (2014): 178–86, doi:10.3746/pnf.2014.19.3.178; M. T. Moradi, M. Rafieian-Kopaei, and A. Karimi, "A Review Study on the Effect of Iranian Herbal Medicines against In Vitro Replication of Herpes simplex Virus," *Avicenna Journal of Phytomedicine* 6, no. 5 (2016): 506–15.

78. Lust, *The Herb Book*, 236–37.

79. "Hyssop, Attractive Flowers and a Great Herbal History," EatThePlanet. org (website), accessed July 28, 2021.

80. Morningbird, "Hyssop: Folklore, Healing & Magickal Uses," *Witchipedia* (website), November 27, 2019.

81. "Ivy," The Eldrum Tree (website), accessed May 8, 2021.

82. Willow, "Magical and Medicinal Uses of Ivy," *Flying the Hedge* (blog), December 16, 2017.

83. Trevor Dines, "Why We Weave Magical Ivy Garlands," BBC Earth (website), December 15, 2015.

84. Folkard, *Plant Lore, Legends, and Lyrics,* 388–91.

85. Rena Goldman, "Everything You Want to Know about English Ivies," Healthline (website), accessed July 29, 2021.

86. D. Hofmann, M. Hecker, and A. Völp, "Efficacy of Dry Extract of Ivy Leaves in Children with Bronchial Asthma—A Review of Randomized Controlled Trials," *Phytomedicine* 10, no. 2–3 (2003): 213–20, doi:10.1078/094471103321659979.

87. Anuradha Rai, "The Anti-inflammatory and Antiarthritic Properties of Ethanol Extract of *Hedera helix*," *Indian Journal of Pharmacological Science* 75, no. 1 (2013): 99–102, doi:10.4103/0250-474X.113537.

88. Lust, *The Herb Book*, 182–83.

89. "English Ivy—Special Precautions and Warnings," WebMD (website), accessed August 2, 2021.

90. Bree NicCarran, "Ivy (*Hedera helix*)," *The Road Goes Ever On* (blog) on Tumblr, accessed July 29, 2021.

91. Anonymous, *Cultus Arborum: A Descriptive Account of Phallic Tree Worship* (privately printed, 1890), 73.

92. Folkard, *Plant Lore, Legends, and Lyrics,* 395.

93. Sarah Corbett, "Juniper Medicine for the Solstice Season," Rowan + Sage (website), accessed August 1, 2021.

94. Folkard, *Plant Lore, Legends, and Lyrics,* 397.

95. "Juniper Mythology and Folklore," Trees for Life (website), accessed July 1, 2021.

96. Lust, *The Herb Book,* 243–44.

97. "Juniper—Special Precautions and Warnings," WebMD (website), accessed August 4, 2021.

98. Morningbird, "Juniper: Folklore, Healing & Magickal Uses," *Witchipedia* (website), November 28, 2019.

99. Gernot Katzer, "Laurel (*Laurus nobilis* L.)," Gernot Katzer's Spice Pages, November 10, 1998.

100. "The Goddess Strenua," *Ancient Romans* (blog) on Tumblr, accessed August 18, 2021.

101. Susan Belsinger, "Bay (*Laurus nobilis*): From Legend and Lore to Fragrance and Flavor," *Fine Gardening* (website), accessed August 9, 2021.

102. Wendy Robbins, "Bay Laurel Essential Oil (Laurel Leaf Essential Oil)," Aromaweb (website), accessed August 9, 2021.

103. "Health Benefits of Bay Laurel—*Laurus nobilis,*" healthbenefitstimes. com (website), accessed August 12, 2021.

104. "Bay Leaf—Special Precautions and Warnings," WebMD (website), accessed August 12, 2021.

105. Vaya, "Bay Leaves (Bay Laurel)," *Information and Correspondents in Witchcraft* (blog) on Tumblr, accessed August 18, 2021.

106. Editore, "The Lemon—the Golden Fruit," Cinqueterre (website), accessed August 19, 2021.

107. Natasha Frost, "In Ancient Rome, Citrus Fruits Were Status Symbols," Atlas Obscura (website), July 25, 2017.

108. "Health and Wellbeing in the Ancient World: 2.2 Citrus Fruits at Pompeii," OpenLearn website of the Open University, accessed August 19, 2021.

109. Marie Josèphe Moncorgé, "Fruit in Medieval Europe," Old Cook (website), accessed August 21, 2021.

110. "The Fruit of Promise: Citrus Fruits in Art and Culture at the Germanisches National Museum," ArtListings (website), May 23, 2011.

111. "History of the Citrus and Citrus Tree Growing in America," Ty Ty Plant Nursery (website), accessed August 21, 2021.

112. "Lemon," RxList (website), accessed August 21, 2021.

113. Lust, *The Herb Book,* 252–53.

114. Megan Ware, "How Can Lemons Benefit Your Health?" Medical News Today (website), November 4, 2019.

115. "How to Use Lemons in Witchcraft 9 Ways," Moody Moons (website), June 30, 2019.

116. "Simply Sweet, A Brief History of Licorice Candy," *Candy Club* (blog), February 11, 2019.

117. Carolina Quaranta, "I·ATE Food Term: Eating Coal in Italy," Terminology Coordination, European Parliament DG Trad (website), June 1, 2018.

118. C. Fiore, M. Eisenhut, E. Ragazzi, et al., "A History of the Therapeutic Use of Liquorice in Europe," *Journal of Ethnopharmacology* 99, no. 3 (2005): 317–24, doi:10.1016/j.jep/2005/04.015.

119. Natalie Silver, "Can You Use Deglycyrrhizinated Licorice (DGL) to Treat Acid Reflux?" Healthline (website), accessed August 24, 2021.

120. Lust, *The Herb Book,* 254–55.

121. "Licorice—Special Precautions and Warnings," WebMD (website), accessed August 24, 2021.

122. "The Monthly Wort: Licorice Root (Part 3)," Mountain Hedgewitch, (website), March 17, 2019.

123. Ladibugs Inc., untitled profile of peppermint, Ladibugs (website), July 2, 2014.

124. Pliny the Elder, "Wild Mint: Twenty Remedies," book 20, chapter 52 of *Natural History,* trans. John Bostock and H. T. Riley (London: Henry G. Bohn, 1855).

125. Ladibugs Inc., untitled profile of peppermint.

126. "How Did Peppermint Become Associated with Christmas?" Askinglot (website), accessed November 8, 2021.

127. Gay Ingram, "Worth a Mint," Homestead.org (website), accessed November 10, 2021.

128. Lust, *The Herb Book,* 275–77.

129. "Peppermint—Side Effects," WebMD (website), accessed November 10, 2021.

130. S. Liddell Macgregor Mathers and George Redway, "Of the Water, and of the Hyssop," chapter 11 of *The Key of Solomon the King, (Clavicula Salomonis)* (London, 1888).

131. "Balder—Loved by Everyone," Historiska (website), accessed August 26, 2021.

132. Pliny the Elder, vol. 3, book 16, chapter 95 of *Natural History,* trans. John Bostock and H. T. Riley (London: Henry G. Bohn, 1855).

133. "Ritual of Oak and Mistletoe," LinkFang (website), accessed August 26, 2021.

134. Ellen Evert Hopman, *Scottish Herbs and Fairy Lore* (Los Angeles: Pendraig Publishing, 2010), 154–55.

135. "European Mistletoe—Side Effects," WebMD (website), accessed August 26, 2021.

136. "Remembering the Magic of Mistletoe," The Hazel Tree (website), December 8, 2019.

137. Linda Lum, "Exploring Nutmeg: Dark History of the Christmas Spice and My Favorite Recipes," Delishably (website), accessed October 25, 2021.

138. Linda Lum, "Exploring Nutmeg."

139. Cora Lin Daniels and C. M. Stevans, *Encyclopædia of Superstitions, Folklore, and the Occult Sciences of the World,* vol. 3 (Honolulu: University Press of the Pacific, 2003), 1500.

140. Jillian Kubala, "8 Science-Backed Benefits of Nutmeg," Healthline (website), accessed October 26, 2021.

141. "Nutmeg," Drugs.com (website), accessed October 26, 2021.

142. Rachel Patterson, "The Magic of Yuletide Spices," Beneath the Moon (website), December 6, 2017.

143. Folkard, *Plant Lore, Legends, and Lyrics,* 468.

144. Folkard, *Plant Lore, Legends, and Lyrics,* 7–8, 22.

145. Ellen Evert Hopman, *A Druid's Herbal of Sacred Tree Medicine* (Rochester, Vt.: Destiny Books, 2008), 56–58.

146. "Oak Bark—Side Effects," RxList (website), accessed November 1, 2021.

147. Hopman, *A Druid's Herbal of Sacred Tree Medicine,* 61.

148. Kelli Foster, "Here's Why We Put Oranges in Stockings at Christmas," Kitchn (website), May 1, 2019.

149. Folkard, *Plant Lore, Legends, and Lyrics,* 477–78.

150. Lust, *The Herb Book,* 298–99.

151. "10 Amazing Health Benefits of Orange Peels," Manipal Hospitals (website), accessed November 3, 2021.

152. A. M. Tacon, "Side Effects of Orange Peel Extract," Leaf (website), accessed November 3, 2021.

153. Racheal Link, "5 Surprising Health Benefits of Orange Juice," Healthline (website), accessed November 3, 2021.

154. Ellen Evert Hopman, *Tree Medicine Tree Magic* (Los Angeles: Pendraig Publishing, 2017), 33–34.

155. Elle Andra-Warner, "The World's First Christmas Tree," *Northern Wilds Magazine* (online), November 27, 2018.

156. Sheri Stritof, "The Bride's Tree: The Symbolism behind the Twelve Ornaments," The Spruce (website), accessed April 16, 2021.

157. Chloe Foussianes, "Queen Victoria and Prince Albert Made Christmas Trees a Holiday Staple," Town & Country (website), December 18, 2018.

158. "The Great Tree of Peace (Skaęhetsiʔkona)," Indigenous Values Initiative, accessed November 11, 2021.

159. Hopman, *Tree Medicine Tree Magic,* 31–32.

160. Lust, *The Herb Book,* 392.

161. "Pine," RxList (website), accessed November 13, 2021.

162. Hopman, *Tree Medicine Tree Magic,* 33–34.

163. Jessika Tucrow, "The Poignant Poinsettia," *My Alchemical Romance* (blog), December 14, 2018.

164. Zack Sterkenberg, "The Long, Strange Tale of the Poinsettia," *Ambius* (blog), December 2, 2019; Judy King, "Christmas Holidays in Mexico: Festivals of Light, Love and Peace," MexConnect (website), accessed November 18, 2021.

165. "Properties of Poinsettia," Botanical Online (website), accessed January 18, 2021; "Poinsettia (Da Ji)," White Rabbit Institute of

Healing, accessed November 18, 2021; "Health Benefits of Poinsettia," healthbenefitstimes.com (website), accessed November 18, 2021.

166. "Poinsettia—Special Precautions and Warnings," WebMD (website), accessed November 18, 2021.

167. Leonard Perry, "Herbs with a Holiday History," University of Vermont Extension Department of Plant and Soil Science, accessed November 21, 2021.

168. Folkard, *Plant Lore, Legends, and Lyrics,* 525–28.

169. Sanford-Burnham Medical Research Institute, "Compound Found in Rosemary Protects Against Macular Degeneration in Laboratory Model," ScienceDaily (website), November 27, 2012.

170. Lust, *The Herb Book,* 338.

171. Joseph Nordqvist, "Everything You Need to Know about Rosemary," Medical News Today (website), December 13, 2017.

172. Paul Beyerl, *A Compendium of Herbal Magick* (Washington: Phoenix Publishing, 1998), 314–16.

173. Patti Wigington, "Rosemary," Learn Religions (website), August 28, 2020.

174. Folkard, *Plant Lore, Legends, and Lyrics,* 44.

175. Suzan Bellincampi, "Star of Bethlehem Is Fleeting Floral Feast," *Vineyard Gazette* (online), June 7, 2018.

176. "Star of Bethlehem Flower—Meaning, Symbolism and Colors," Flower Meanings (website), accessed November 26, 2021.

177. "Star of Bethlehem—Special Precautions and Warnings," WebMD (website), accessed November 27, 2021.

178. "Striking Facts about the Star of Bethlehem Flower," Gardenerdy (website), accessed November 26, 2021.

179. Edward Bach, M.D., *The Twelve Healers and Other Remedies,* as quoted in "Star of Bethlehem," Bach Centre (website), accessed November 27, 2021.

180. "#35 Star of Bethlehem Flower Meaning & Symbolism," TreeSymbolism .com (website), accessed November 27, 2021.

181. Robininscarf, "Star of Bethlehem Roots Sauteed with Onions and Scrambled Eggs," post on Reddit (website), accessed November 27, 2021.

182. Diane Kochilas, "Horta-Greens: A Glossary of Edible Wild Greens," personal blog, January 1, 2020.

183. Patricia Rain, "History of Vanilla," The Vanilla Company (website), February 26, 2009.

184. Vivien Lee, "The Epic, Sensational, Anything-But-Plain Story of Vanilla," Thrillist.com (website), September 18, 2017.

185. Anders, "Vanilla! Vanilla!" IceCreamNation.org (website), December 10, 2011.

186. "Vanilla," RxList (website), accessed December 8, 2021.

187. Andrea Boldt, "What Are the Health Benefits of Vanilla Extract?" Livestrong.com (website), August 26, 2019.

188. Lizzie Ball, "Eight Surprising Health Benefits of Vanilla," *Salt of the Earth* (blog), August 22, 2018.

189. Amaria, "Be Inspired by the Magickal Properties of Vanilla," Wicca Now (website), accessed December 8, 2021.

Index of Recipes
and Projects

Recipes

Projects

Index of Plants
by Common Name

Numbers in *italics* preceded by *pl.* refer to color insert plate numbers.

298

Index of Plants
by Scientific Name

Numbers in *italics* preceded by *pl.* refer to color insert plate numbers.

General Index

Numbers in *italics* preceded by *pl.* refer to color insert plate numbers.

Books of Related Interest

The Sacred Herbs of Samhain
Plants to Contact the Spirits of the Dead
by Ellen Evert Hopman
Foreword by Andrew Theitic

The Sacred Herbs of Spring
Magical, Healing, and Edible Plants to Celebrate Beltaine
by Ellen Evert Hopman

Secret Medicines from Your Garden
Plants for Healing, Spirituality, and Magic
by Ellen Evert Hopman

A Druid's Herbal for the Sacred Earth Year
by Ellen Evert Hopman

A Druid's Herbal of Sacred Tree Medicine
by Ellen Evert Hopman

Once Around the Sun
Stories, Crafts, and Recipes to Celebrate the Sacred Earth Year
by Ellen Evert Hopman
Illustrated by Lauren Mills
Foreword by Jane Yolen

Walking the World in Wonder
by Ellen Evert Hopman

The Real Witches of New England
History, Lore, and Modern Practice
by Ellen Evert Hopman
Foreword by Judika Illes

INNER TRADITIONS • BEAR & COMPANY
P.O. Box 388
Rochester, VT 05767
1-800-246-8648 • www.InnerTraditions.com

Or contact your local bookseller